ADVANCE PRAISE

"Aggie is an inspiring force of nature. In Biohack Like a Woman, *she guides you on a path to reveal and realize more of your limitless potential."*

–Jim Kwik,
World's leading brain coach &
NYT bestselling author of *Limitless*

"Biohack Like a Woman? *More like 'Game Changer'! Aggie Lal's refreshing take on biology puts women's health back in the driver's seat. It's about time for women to own their power. So grateful for this invaluable knowledge and inspiration."*

–Ricki Lake,
TV personality, host of The Ricki Lake Show,
and producer of *"The Business of Being Born,"*

"Biohack Like a Woman *is a testament to Lal's pioneering efforts to redefine biohacking for women. It will be an invaluable tool for any female seeking self-betterment."*

–Daniel G. Amen, MD,
Double-Board Psychiatrist & 12-time
New York Times bestselling author

"I knew. Straight away. Aggie is truly a bestie. To me. To women. To young girls. She's inspiring, passionate, and on a mission to make everyone around her healthier and happier."

–Shawn Wells, MPH, RD, LDN, CISSN, FISSN,
World's Greatest Formulator &
bestselling author of *The ENERGY Formula*

"*Aggie has created an essential guide that brilliantly bridges the gap between cutting-edge science and everyday wellness. A must-read for any woman looking to elevate their health and therefore happiness through innovative and proven techniques.*"

–Emily Fletcher,
Founder of Ziva Meditation &
bestselling author of *Stress Less, Accomplish More*

BIOHACK
LIKE A WOMAN

How to Get Fit Effortlessly,
Feel Beautiful, Have More
Energy, and Unleash
Your Superpowers
With Biohacking

AGGIE LAL

BIOHACK **LIKE A WOMAN**
How to Get Fit Effortlessly, Feel Beautiful, Have More Energy, and Unleash Your Superpowers With Biohacking

For permission requests, speaking inquiries, and bulk order purchase options, email aggie@biohackingbestie.com.

Biohacking Bestie
25 FIRST AVE SW, STE A, WATERTOWN, SD 57201

http://biohacklikeawoman.com

Designed by Transcendent Publishing | TranscendentPublishing.com
Edited by Tiffany Brooks
Copy Edited by Mary Rembert
Cover photography by Jacob Riglin
Secondary photography: Anna Mioduszewska

ISBN: 979-8-9896548-0-2

DISCLAIMER
I make a lot of recommendations and share observations from other biohacking experts, but before you implement any advice you're about to read, you need to consult with your health practitioner. It can be hard to find someone who shares a similar outlook on food, but ask about tests you can run before, during, and after modifying your lifestyle to find out what's working and what's not. That way, you'll know what to keep, what to tweak, and what to toss. Remember, there's no such thing as a one-size-fits-all approach when it comes to biohacking.

Printed in the United States of America

For my biohacking sisters

The more women who step into their power,
the more sisters I get to share adventures with.

Kiki, this one is for you.

To Be a Woman

I learned to be a woman
by how the world raised me.

Be silent, it said.
So I spoke.

Be weak, it whispered.
So I grew.

Sit down, it said.
So I stood.

What it means to be a woman
is to be told to be nothing …

And become everything.

— Unknown

CONTENTS

FOREWORD

In 2011, I started the biohacking movement with a blog post and started the first biohacking conference, which was only 100 people in a bar in San Francisco, and about 80% were men. Within a year of that first blog post, 60% of the biohackers were women. As I grew my company, Bulletproof, to become a major new disruptive force in creating healthy food, women made up the ranks of customers more often than men.

In 2018, Merriam-Webster added biohacking to the list of new words in the English language. I defined it as "The art and science of changing the environment around you and inside of you so you have full control of your own biology."

It has since become a global movement, with biohackers in every country doing whatever it takes to have the energy and the type of life they want. And the truth is, women often take to biohacking more easily than men! When I brought up this observation with women in my life, they laughed at me and said, "That's because our bodies change just about every day, and you guys don't notice anything is wrong unless a bone is sticking out."

And therein lies the rub: women may be better at noticing changes, but they have to deal with more of them. It is frustrating that most medical studies until the last decade often excluded women because of these types of changes. So, the principles of biohacking apply to all humans, and I go out of my way to include all of the studies I can find that are specific to women, but there is a lack of information.

And that is why I am thrilled to introduce you to Aggie and her groundbreaking book, *Biohack Like a Woman*, which shines a light on biohacking for women. This book isn't just informative; it's a guide that empowers and is especially designed for women.

Biohacking isn't supposed to be intimidating. Aggie demystifies this by providing clear, practical, and achievable strategies. These strategies are not just theoretical ideals; they are born from her own experiences and the collective wisdom of the biohacking community. In *Biohack Like a Woman*, Aggie teaches women to become architects of their own health, providing them with the tools and knowledge to navigate the biohacking landscape confidently.

In fact, most often biohacking validates ancestral knowledge that was often handed down from our grandmothers and their grandmothers. It represents a science-based way to reintroduce us to our heritage, in which we are responsible for our own health and for that of the community around us, both men and women. It's exciting that we have more information than ever before, and we have a much greater ability to change the environment around us to improve our energy, our mood, and just about every aspect of our lives.

Aggie's foray into biohacking stemmed from her own health challenges and the demands of a career that required extensive travel. Realizing the need to take charge of her biology for a better quality of life, she began exploring the world of biohacking. Her journey led her to attend my Biohacking Conference, which now hosts about 3,000 vibrant humans coming together to figure out new biohacking ideas and to learn from each other. That's where I met Aggie for the first time! I've since been on her podcast several times, and she on mine.

She goes deep, though—spending countless time at Upgrade Labs, my biohacking franchise that is opening doors across North America, and even going deep into her own brain at my brain biohacking facility called 40 Years of Zen. She documented her journey there online and inspired so many women to understand that the psychological, emotional, and even spiritual parts of you are things you can change. It's been so much fun to spend time with Aggie, as she has chosen to use biohacking to rapidly evolve and improve herself in so many ways.

I like Aggie's approach in *Biohack Like a Woman* because she offers strategies that are easy to start and adaptable to individual needs. Her work is particularly pioneering for women. The hustle and grind culture that made me burn out before I was 30 is even more toxic for women, who generally require a greater focus on recovery and stress management to support their unique biology. Yet one of the most frustrating aspects of the health and fitness movement is that it is encouraging everyone to burn themselves out while starving on a low-calorie diet. As veteran biohackers have probably heard, both men and women will hit the wall, but women, on average, will hit it first because of hormonal differences. Aggie is all over this and makes it safe and accessible to focus on recovery as a performance and quality-of-life activity. I love it.

If you saw just one "biohacker bro" site, you'd be tempted to say biohacking is male-dominated, but it cannot be. That's because the most important part of the environment around you (after air and water, maybe) is your community. And your community is composed of men and women. When a woman chooses to improve her health and well-being, everyone around her benefits. And vice versa. You can see this in Aggie's own life as she took control of her health and her energy and documented it on her social media platforms.

Aggie's work in *Biohack Like a Woman* addresses this by customizing biohacking strategies to meet the unique physiological and lifestyle needs of women. She provides a nuanced and holistic approach, contrasting with traditional health and fitness regimes that often push individuals to extreme limits. Aggie emphasizes the importance of recovery, a principle I've always advocated in biohacking, even though the message often doesn't land until you burn out. When you read this book, Aggie's message will land!

One significant aspect that Aggie brings to light is the additional challenges women face around toxins. Mainstream lifestyles expose women to more toxins, particularly through products like makeup and skincare. Aggie's deep understanding of these unique challenges places women as equal partners in the biohacking journey. And women face more pressure to eat exactly the diets that create stress: those without enough calories or nutrients.

Biohack Like a Woman is more than a book; it's an important part of growing the biohacking movement. It offers women practical, achievable blueprints to follow, embodying the capacity for self-empowerment and betterment. This book is the first of its kind, designed specifically with women in mind, and explores the intricate and beautiful universe of biohacking for women through solid scientific research and practical advice.

What sets *Biohack Like a Woman* apart is Aggie's balanced approach to biohacking. She navigates away from the extremes often seen in traditional health and fitness, focusing instead on a sustainable, holistic path. This balance between pushing the limits and prioritizing recovery is critical, especially for women who juggle multiple roles in today's fast-paced world. Aggie's insights offer a way to achieve optimal health without compromising other aspects of life.

Aggie's impact through *Biohack Like a Woman* goes beyond individual health. By gifting women with the knowledge and tools for biohacking, she's creating a ripple effect that extends to families, communities, and even broader society. As more women embrace biohacking, they become role models, inspiring others around them to prioritize their health and well-being. There's nothing like seeing a happy, healthy, vibrant person literally skipping down the street to lift you from whatever raw, kale-fueled doldrum you may be caught in. If you don't believe it, come to The Biohacking Conference and hang out with Aggie and me!

Biohack Like a Woman is more than a book; it's a call to action. It invites women to engage actively with their health, to question conventional wisdom, and to explore new possibilities in wellness. Aggie's work is a testament to the power of biohacking in transforming lives, and it encourages women to take the first step on this empowering journey.

As I endorse *Biohack Like a Woman*, I do so with the belief that this book will mark a significant milestone in the biohacking community. Aggie's work is a beacon of hope and a guide for women, inspiring them to take control of their health and unlock their full potential. It's an honor to support Aggie's vision, one that aligns so closely with my own—to make biohacking an easy, widely available transformative tool for all.

With gratitude,
Dave Asprey,
CEO, Upgrade Labs, 40 Years of Zen, and Danger Coffee

INTRODUCTION

Picture this: I'm Aggie Lal, a travel influencer known to my million followers as Travel in Her Shoes. Even though I spent 300 days a year taking photos in the dreamiest locations (Bora Bora, Bali, Barcelona—you name it!), truly living the dream, I realized a few years ago that I needed to make some serious changes to my hard-core vegan lifestyle. I was sipping kale smoothies and oat milk lattes—all the things that were supposed to make me glowing, gorgeous, and healthy—and I was exhausted.

At first, I chalked it up to traveling. Time zones can jack with your sleep and circadian rhythms, so that was probably it, right? Besides, everyone is tired. We're all chugging a couple of cups of coffee to make it through the day.

Then came the bloating that made my stomach stick out like I was six months pregnant—which would have been great if I had, you know, *actually been six months pregnant*. But I wasn't. This was followed by weight gain that snuck up like a ninja and mood swings I couldn't control.

Then the depression, followed by pimples and hair loss—in patches! *Cool.* Sure, I was successful, but you can't filter fatigue and sadness. You can't Photoshop the energy you wish you had into your real life. Something had to change, and fast.

I was blessed to have the funds and the access to consult the best doctors in New York City, and, boy, the time I spent in the doctor's office. Imagine burning through $20,000 on tests and treatments that give you hope one minute and another dead-end the next. I felt confused and hopeless. Are there pills for bloating and exhaustion? Sure, but it felt like one solution brought three side effects. This was not sustainable, nor was it me. I embraced an organic, holistic life-style. Loading up on manufactured pharmaceuticals felt counter-productive to living my best life.

Finally, out of sheer desperation to try something—anything—I stumbled into biohacking. To be more accurate, I crash-landed into it. But I landed in a man's world. Fast for 20 hours a day, cold plunge, and push yourself at the gym. Tag every workout #NoDaysOff. It was … intense. But I was determined, so I charged in head first. Keto? Tried it. Fasting? You bet. No sugar for a month? Yep. But guess what? I was still exhausted, and now I was miserable to boot.

That's why I went rogue and discovered that biohacking for women is a whole other world (and a virtually uninhabited one, at that). There were hardly any other women in this space at the time. Oh, there were plenty of women biohackers, but they were following the process designed for male bodies. Through a lot of trial and almost as much error, I learned what worked and what didn't the hard way so you wouldn't have to. The endgame is this book, *Biohack Like a Woman*, which is all about biohacks tailored for women and written to women by women. This is a hard-fought study of how to make biohacking an empowering and exciting path toward your own health goals.

This is how you become a biohacker—yes, *you*. The gorgeous woman reading this right now who wishes she had the discipline and drive to become a biohacker, but who also has that annoying thing called "real life" that's always breathing down her neck.

I put all those golden nuggets into a single book that cuts through the noise. Imagine a world where you *don't* have to sift through 200 books, podcasts, and questionable Reddit threads. We're talking about a curated, no-BS guide to reclaiming your health and vitality in a way that will change your life without dominating it. *Biohack Like a Woman* is your fast track to a new you: energized, confident, and as radiant as the morning sun over a Bali beach—no filters needed.

Are you ready to ditch the guesswork and go straight for the life-altering, soul-shaking truths? *Biohack like a Woman* is your roadmap to a life less ordinary. The transformation you've been waiting for is just a page-turn away. Ready to dive in?

Now, I get that you might be asking why I wrote my own book on biohacking instead of sending you to the titans in this space. Well, a lot of them don't have ovaries (not that ovaries define a woman, but I think you catch my drift). Dave Asprey is the father of biohacking, and I am … your bestie. Your biohacking bestie. With ovaries—and a different perspective on the whole thing as a result.

As your bestie, I know you have a million things going on. New job? Break up? Baby on the way? Situationship? It's all so much. Adding another thing onto your plate—learning the science of biohacking— can be overwhelming. And I don't want you to give up on yourself because of lack of time or because your body isn't responding the way you hoped and dreamed it would.

The thing is, I want you to feel your best—or if that's too much to think about right now with everything else happening in your life, let's just go with "better." I want you to feel *better* than you do right now.

And here's how we are going to make that happen: My superpower is translating complicated medical research (with a group of scientists on my team) into super simple, bite-sized (pun intended) bits of information that you can digest while living your busy life, whether you are reading this book on the train to the office, waiting in the pickup line at your kid's school, or walking your pet. I am translating the research not because I don't think you're smart enough to understand it but because I see you, and I know that you are juggling a million things in life.

This book supports women who support everyone else.

I'll also share my personal journey from being a vegan to a hard-core biohacker to now being a mix of a biohacker and a bio-slacker. And I've never been healthier *or* happier. (For real.) Let's get started!

ADOPT THE IDENTITY
OF A BIOHACKER

CHAPTER 1

WHAT IS A BIOHACKER?

By the time Lara (now in her late 20s) turned 18, she was sick all the time. As a young girl, Lara was underweight, so her pediatrician suspected an eating disorder and told her mom to give her any foods she wanted as long as she gained weight.

So, of course, Lara gravitated to junk food—what kid wouldn't if they had the chance? She was the only kid at school with ten packages of cookies for lunch. She'd come home and heat up a frozen cheese pizza with extra melted cheese as a snack. After dinner with her family, there was always dessert because her uncle was a pastry chef. She was eating a ton of sugary foods every day, so she was getting plenty of (empty) calories, but she was still having trouble gaining weight.

Lara eventually developed pneumonia, asthma, and chronic sinusitis. Her doctors kept looking at her lungs but couldn't find anything. It took almost two years to figure out that she had an issue with her tonsils, but her doctor at the time said removal wasn't recommended anymore. Instead, he prescribed antibiotics for a year and a half! Every month, she would get a new box. At one point, she was taking five to ten prescription medications a day.

Lara knows now that being given monthly antibiotics for 18 months was ridiculous, but back then, she didn't know what she didn't know. All she heard was, "Get better, Lara. Just eat more and rest more."

Nobody told her to eat better.

Nobody told her to focus on diet.

Nobody told her to focus on nutrition.

Nobody told her to take probiotics.

Eventually, she started having all kinds of issues with her gut. She had acne, IBS, and chronic migraines. She couldn't handle wearing pants because they felt too tight. Nothing could touch her belly because it was so bloated and painful.

Her symptoms got so severe that her doctor finally told her she might have the beginnings of Crohn's disease. Thankfully, a colonoscopy eventually ruled that out, but something wasn't right.

Her doctor had run all the tests he knew to run, but he wasn't finding any problems his solutions could fix. After five years of trying to get to the root cause of all of her health issues, he finally gave up and said there was nothing else he could do.

But Lara couldn't continue to suffer in pain.

She had already tried all the diets, including gluten-free, lactose-free, and low-FODMAP, but they didn't work for her. Then, she found the GAPS diet, also known as the bone broth diet. It wasn't just drinking bone broth; it was removing processed and inflammatory foods and eating more meat, fish, eggs, and cooked veggies. She found that the only thing she could digest was the meat and bone broth because her gut was so wrecked. But that wasn't enough to sustain her, let alone allow her body to thrive.

Now a woman in her 20s with a career as a scientist, Lara began to do some research on herself. As she was looking into alternatives online, she found my Biohacking Bestie fitness challenge.

I have lots of resources and other specialists to follow that I share as part of the challenge, so Lara started diving into all the biohacking books I recommended. She was so desperate that she tried everything, including taking a DNA test I mentioned. When she did, she learned she had a lower genetic capability of detoxifying her body.

When I mentioned in the challenge that some people can't digest certain anti-nutrients called lectins, Lara noticed that the veggies she had been trying to eat were high in them. She started avoiding those and tried other veggies, and that worked.

She also embraced the importance of balancing her glucose levels for her health. This was a big change for me, and Lara found that it helped her get rid of her terrible junk food cravings that sometimes even led her to eat a bag of chips as dinner.

Later, she found out she had a parasite, so she took some natural remedies to get rid of it, as well. Over the course of about six months, she was able to reverse her IBS and get off the meds. *All of them.*

She had had chronic sinusitis that required a strong nasal spray for years, but she was able to stop taking it. Her chronic migraines went away. She had really bad rosacea on her face that heavy makeup couldn't cover, but she biohacked her results, so even the redness disappeared.

She says that her journey to better gut health was complex, but now she listens more and more to her body. She has found that fasting according to her cycle works really well for her, along with drinking bulletproof coffee, which is Dave Asprey's recipe for coffee with butter and MCT oil (yep, butter in coffee, you read that right!).

She took her health into her own hands so she could finally get to the root of her symptoms, heal from the inside out, and live her best life.

Today, Lara is one of the healthiest and most high-functioning women I know. She says that the Biohacking Bestie community had a huge impact on pointing her toward the right people at the right time.

And the best gift? Lara now serves as part of my research team to help thousands of other women find solutions that are specific to their problems, not just blindly accepting someone's advice.

Lara is the perfect definition of a biohacker. She didn't spend hours each day in the gym or doing cold plunges. She didn't make herself miserable to feel better. But she absolutely changed her life.

What Is Biohacking?

Biohackers are just a bunch of people who love feeling amazing and hate feeling like crap—which, you have to admit, is a pretty solid philosophy for life. So they figured out how to build a lifestyle that keeps them feeling that way by relying on their body's natural or science-backed processes rather than medications or other artificial methods.

Biohacking was and is mostly male-dominated. When I first got into it five years ago, I couldn't find a single female role model I wanted to learn more about or even just grab coffee with. So I followed the big dudes who fasted 20 hours a day, did HIIT training every workout, and cold-plunged daily. The harder they biohacked, the better. It took me too long to realize that our journeys and goals aren't the same, and I simply can't take their advice. In fact, I should think twice before taking advice from anyone who isn't a woman.

"Bikini medicine" is a term for when medicine approaches women's health in the same way as men except in the areas of the body covered by a bikini. Unfortunately, bikini biohacking is very much a thing.

Bikini biohacking assumes women's biohacking should be the same as men's, minus the bikini areas. In fact, we manage stress differently, we sleep differently, we eat differently.

After coaching almost 20,000 women, I know we are not just smaller, less hairy versions of men. (I mean, I knew that *before* coaching 20,000 women, but working with that many ladies confirmed it.) On top of that, I have come to believe that women are more natural biohackers than men are. We are inherently more connected to our intuition, bodies, nutrition, and self-care. We have a long history of tuning into our bodies due to the complexities of our cycles, pregnancy, and motherhood. Historically, it is women who have been herbalists and healers. Women were the people we trusted with our health. Women carried life and they sustained life. We are naturally *really good* at this. Women were doing science for millennia before science was even a thing.

Think about it: our monthly cycle is a kind of built-in biofeedback mechanism that makes women more attuned to subtle changes in their bodies, energy levels, and cravings. It gives us an incredible advantage over men in understanding what our body needs in terms of constantly adjusting and "hacking" various aspects of our life, from diet and exercise to stress management and sleep during our menstrual cycle. And we do most of this without even thinking about it, which arguably makes us more nimble and innovative biohackers when we attempt to do it more deliberately because we've already been doing some version of this for years!

Now, I understand that not all women have regular periods for a variety of reasons. And I've seen a lot of fitness trainers who might look fit but struggle with endometriosis, polycystic ovarian syndrome (PCOS), or no period at all. The thing is, your period is your fifth vital sign, so if it's missing or not showing up in the healthiest way possible, it may be time to adjust your diet and lifestyle.

Unfortunately, so much of our natural power has been outsourced in this modern world of ours—outsourced to medicine, social demands, cultural pressures, and every other external force that we are expected to bow down to instead of listening to our own beautiful, brilliant bodies and the wisdom they still carry.

I know it's an unpopular opinion in the medical realm that something as simple as "only" changes to diet, lifestyle, and environment can heal you. But isn't it diet, environment, and lifestyle that created the "dis-ease" in your body in the first place?

Pills, intricate diet plans, and everything else that promises to "fix your life" usually come with a cost—both in terms of long-term damage to your body as well as actual cash. But biohacking only requires a few mindset shifts, some new daily practices, and maybe a tweak or two to your daily routine. What other system can you think of that allows you to level up in life, health, and overall well-being … without costing you a cent?

I am going to be completely honest with you: Biohacking can get expensive—like, really, *really* expensive. We're talking cutting-edge science here that isn't exactly backed by Big Pharma. The costs for various programs, gadgets, supplements, and treatments can quickly add up. In fact, it can feel a lot like golf, dominated by rich white dudes.

And maybe that's been one of the things keeping you from exploring it until now. (The cost, I mean, not all the rich white dudes. But maybe also all the rich white dudes.) But the way I teach biohacking is different. I want to show you that even small adjustments to your lifestyle that don't require you to spend *any money* will make a massive difference. And if later on you want to spend all the money you didn't spend on biohacking on something else, go for it. I am a great shopping buddy! Take me with you. But we aren't spending any money on biohacking unless you just really want to.

Everything I am sharing with you in this book is relatively free. Now, would gadgets and supplements make it easier for you? Sure. As a founder of a supplement company, I am obsessed with using the "shortcuts" nutritional supplements offer that are otherwise not available in our food and water. But my goal here isn't to push my products. (I mention a few, but nothing I describe depends on using them). My goal is to empower you as a woman because that's supposedly what good feminists are supposed to do: We support other women. We have each other's backs. We cheer each other on rather than tear each other down.

Well, I am a good feminist, and I am cheering my head off for you. I can't wait to see where this journey takes you.

An Overwhelmed Woman Doesn't Biohack

Biohacking is a process; it's not 1s and 0s. It gives you a choice. Don't let anyone shame you for "still" using or doing something. Remember, we live in a free-will universe; you've *always* got a choice. My role here is to arm you with information because awareness gives you freedom to make those decisions consciously. After all, doing something out of a lack of awareness isn't really choosing—it's being manipulated. It's very different to take a birth control pill thinking it has no side effects vs. *choosing* to take it for your current circumstances with full awareness of what it does so that when you do notice side effects, you can respond accordingly.

I've noticed many women don't get into biohacking, fearing it's too black and white, with intense and rigid rules that will require them to give up their favorite makeup or Botox or whatever. My approach is not about getting everything perfect but making small changes toward what's doable *now*. There is a saying that "a confused customer doesn't buy," and I think it's also true that "an overwhelmed woman doesn't biohack." Following strict rules can make a woman feel dominated—and not in any kind of good way.

Mainstream diet and lifestyle gurus tell you to eat small meals throughout the day and snack more; on the other extreme, the hardcore biohackers tell you to fast 20 hours a day and pack an entire day's worth of calories into the remaining four.

How about—oh, I don't know—maybe trusting your own body to tell you how and in what way she needs to be nourished?

The problem with most diets is that they assume you're not smart enough to understand the science behind the advice (*maybe because there isn't any or else it's outdated information from the 1980s*) and too disconnected from your gut feeling to trust your intuition of knowing what's best for your body.

And most of the science you'll find on how to get healthy or lose weight quickly is geared toward men because male bodies tend to process calories differently, often resulting in a much easier time losing weight. They can restrict calories, do intermittent fasting for 20 hours a day, and be just fine.

But for women—you know, the ones who are *literally biologically designed to keep the species alive*—any prolonged calorie restriction or any lifestyle that pushes us too much and makes us feel "unsafe" can result in the body holding onto weight, which can lead to massive hormone imbalances and even infertility.

It makes sense, if you think about it. If your body goes into starvation mode, what signal is it receiving from its environment? *It's not safe to get pregnant now. It's not safe for a baby to come into this world because there is not enough food for the mama to keep the pregnancy healthy and not enough food for the baby once it arrives.* Your body is brilliant. It creates all these natural contraceptive mechanisms to make sure the little human doesn't go hungry. It's doing exactly what it is supposed to do: protecting you and any future humans you might grow.

My goal is for women to take extreme ownership of their actions and realize that it is their priority and responsibility to learn about what's best for their bodies to honor and celebrate this incredible machine that you've been given in which to experience life. That includes trusting your gut and listening to—not fighting—the feedback your body is designed to give you.

Biohacking is a tool, not an end in itself. The second that diet or habit makes your life worse, it's no longer wellness. Biohacking isn't one single set of behaviors or practices; it is a curated collection of practices that help you thrive physically, emotionally, and spiritually in your best and healthiest life—whatever that means to you. It's important to understand that bodies are not "one size fits all." Literally.

I really want you to be aware of your degree of choice and agency in this process. When I do self-growth courses with women, I ask them to pay attention to the words they use. For example, I encourage them not to say, "I can't afford this"; instead, I suggest saying, "This is not my priority right now." It's not only more empowering but also more accurate.

In the same way, if your diet isn't super healthy, perhaps it's fair to say it hasn't been your priority lately. Or maybe you are so overworked and tired you can't imagine learning yet another new thing. Either way, give yourself some grace and kindness, and if a few of the suggestions below resonate, great! If you can't make any of them happen, don't worry about it! Stick to Stage 1 for another month or two or another year, if that's realistic. Your call. I'll be here when you're ready.

Put simply, biohacking is self-experimentation on a personal level, so you get to learn what's best for your body. It's following the latest science to optimize your body for the healthiest, strongest you. And it's the opposite of the one-size-fits-all approach to health and wellness.

> **Biohacking:** (verb, noun) (v): To change the environment outside of you and inside of you so you are intimately in tune with your biology to allow you to upgrade your body, mind, and life. (n): The art and science of becoming superhuman.

In other words, biohacking isn't about sticking strictly with one particular diet or a specific set of supplements; it's about using science and technology to make your body function better and more efficiently. It is self-experimentation on a personal level, so you can decide what is best for your body.

That's why we won't be focusing on nitpicking your food choices. Instead, we will dive into why you might be struggling in the first place, how to optimize your lifestyle by syncing it to your menstrual cycle, and loving every part of you so that you can finally step into your main character's energy and become the absolute best version of you.

This means …

1. Taking FULL responsibility for your health. This is the first key to being your own bestie who loves, listens to, protects, and nurtures herself. You owe yourself accountability; and

2. Being flexible to self-experimenting, testing what makes your body feel good and what makes your body feel sick, and adapting as needed.

BIOHACKING

B: Biology

We understand that changing biology changes our state, our mind, and our life. And we start changing our life by feeling better so we can be better, do better, and make the world a better place.

I: Individuality

(The "I" factor). We understand that everyone is different, and we only have about 10% of our gut in common, so a diet or biohack that works for me might not work for you.

O: Optimization

You are committed to making the best and most effective and efficient use of your situation or resources available to get the results (health and energy).

H: Health

This is the #1 value in biohacking. Health is true wealth. Healthy is the new sexy. We don't do things for looks; we do them to nourish our bodies and to be healthy and strong. And also to age in reverse.

A: Attention to Details

Details make a huge difference. The nuances of each bit of advice are very important. Small details matter, so pay attention to micro adjustments.

C: Community and Culture

Biohacking is an incredible, supportive, and fun community. We're here to support each other. We know that people who live in communities are happier and live longer.

K: Knowledge

We base our advice and lives on the latest science, and we check sources that can be looked up and confirmed on verified, public websites like PubMed.gov.

I: Intuition
Trust in your body's natural intelligence instead of dismissing it.

N: Never Stop Learning
We read books like this one, listen to podcasts (like *Biohacking Bestie*!), attend seminars, and stay curious.

G: Get to the Root
We understand that symptoms are our body's signals, so instead of treating symptoms, we search for the root cause (glucose spikes, for example). Biohacking isn't anti-medicine. Biohacking is *the gap between* dieting and medicine.

Most diets aren't based on the latest science. In conducting research for this book and my biohacking podcast, I lovingly and probably a little obsessively stalked the popular information out there right now. I was curious about what was being said by the leaders in the dieting industry, and what I found depressed me.

These nutrition myths are still being spread far and wide:

- All calories are the same, and you should count them.
- Fat makes you fat.
- Snacks are great—always carry nuts and fruit with you.
- Have five to six meals a day.
- Smoothies and juices are the way to go.
- Eat your dessert before your meal to lose weight.
- Vegan alternatives are better than the real thing (like grass-fed butter).
- Drop red meat and have lean chicken breast instead. (My mouth feels dry as I write this!)

No wonder our collective health is getting worse instead of better!

I went to one fitness page with four million followers that I found online because I figured she must be doing something right.

Smiling serenely back at me from the landing page is a beautiful woman with great genetics and an indented stomach. She suggests her favorite breakfast smoothie: oat milk, a banana, two spoons of brown sugar that can be replaced with a date, and her brand of protein powder.

Three hours later, I can have juice and rice crackers with almond butter. Dang. It sure does look Instagrammy.

Continuing to the next page of this site, she makes more suggestions: a mozzarella sandwich for breakfast, a smoothie for a snack, then spaghetti bolognese for lunch. I follow this diet for half a day, checking my glucose levels with my CGM (continuous glucose monitor). Instead of my body launching into blissful appreciation for all this lovely nourishment I'm giving it, my glucose spikes are off the charts. By 2 p.m., all I want is carbs and sugar, even though my body needs protein and healthy fats.

For me and 95% of women, this meal plan will create massive glucose spikes throughout the day. Glucose spikes lead to hormone imbalance, saggy skin, cellulite, bloating, fatigue, general bitchiness, more cravings, and gut issues. And years and years of glucose spikes lead to preventable (but often terminal) diseases.

No wonder women feel like there is something wrong with them when eating like this and not seeing results. The misinformation is paralyzing. The worst part is you can find proof that any diet works because it probably did for someone somewhere, probably in a highly curated environment designed to maximize their biological predisposition for this kind of approach.

The truth is that just by cutting calories, any diet can make you lose weight temporarily. It's also relatively easy to see results for someone who has never paid attention to their fitness level and now starts watching what they eat and moving their body because any kind of activity and thoughtful eating will give some sort of yield.

But, most likely, neither of those women are you. You know exercise matters. You know you should be eating the way you want to feel. And you certainly don't live in a custom-curated environment where all your stress is removed, your calendar is clear for working out whenever you feel like it, and someone is taking care of all the grocery shopping, meal prep, and clean-up. (If you *do* live that life, give me a call. I want to learn your secret.)

But why should you trust me to offer advice for *your* body any more than you should trust whatever lifestyle and diet influencer is currently dominating social media at the moment with tips and recipes to help you make your life look just like hers? Because I'm not trying to tell you how to replicate *my* life; I'm trying to empower you to maximize *your own*.

Who Is Aggie Lal? (Hint: It's Me!)

Before I became one of the first female biohackers and did things like create courses (that now serve thousands of women all over the world), and start a podcast where I interview legends like Wim Hof and Glennon Doyle, and speak on stages with experts like Dave Asprey and Jim Kwik, and start my own Biohacking Bestie supplement line with renowned biochemist and formulator Shawn Wells—before I did all that, I was a hard-core calorie-counting, oat milk-drinking, fat-avoiding vegan whose health had started going to hell.

But my health journey actually starts even earlier than that. I began "dieting" when I was 12 years old. My Polish mom would make me ham and cheese sandwiches for breakfast or Polish sausage, and I was called "Little Pasta," "Meatball," and "Dumpling" growing up because I was pudgy. I watched my plate sizing with every meal and lived in constant dread of fat for another ten years until I moved to LA and started working in the film business. There, I learned that every woman around me seemed to have three things in common: she had her boobs done, she did yoga, and she was vegan.

I was already doing yoga, so I figured that I should give a vegan diet a try (and the boobs!). It resonated with me on so many levels because I couldn't bring myself to eat animals anymore. And as I dropped weight (down to 89 pounds, in fact), my vegan ego grew. It became my identity, and I was obsessed with this new, smarter, and thinner me who was so much better than the old, non-vegan me. I would have ten meals a day and absolutely no metabolic flexibility (you will learn what that is later in the book), but I convinced myself that didn't matter because "the skinnier, the better" was the mantra I believed in more than I ever believed in myself and my health, nutrition, overall well-being, and inherent value.

In 2016, I was waiting for my green card to get approved and was unemployed for six months, but I wasn't partying or sunbathing all day. Not at all. I would wake up at 5:55 every morning and go to the gym to walk on a treadmill for an hour while listening to motivational videos. I was far from home and family, and I missed having people around me who inspired me every day, so instead I hung out with Tony Robbins's voice on the treadmill each morning.

One of those days on the treadmill, I came across Dave Asprey, who was called "the father of biohacking." Immediately, I tried implementing his advice. I did everything he preached with one small modification: I was still a full-on vegan.

While that was far from what he recommended, I thought I could do it because the first vegan cheeses, butters, and ice cream were starting to enter the market, and, of course, they seemed so exciting. I would proudly buy all of them because I automatically believed that meant they were better for me and that being vegan was the *only* right path toward better health.

I mean, okay. Sure. Maybe I was starting to bloat a little, and maybe I started noticing a few small pimples and extra breakage in my hair. And then *maybe* the bloating got worse, and the weight started to creep back on, and my face erupted into all-out acne, and my hair was falling out in clumps, and I was developing bald patches. But that's *totally normal* for a fit young woman in her 20s living her healthiest life, right?

By the time I turned 30, I couldn't stand to look at myself in the mirror anymore. I was convinced it was all over, and I would never have smooth skin or a full head of shiny hair again. I spent thousands of dollars on all the best moisturizers, wrinkle treatments, and hair extenders. I was so thoroughly brainwashed into believing that fat would make me fat and that meat was the enemy that I never stopped to question whether being vegan was, in fact, not the healthiest choice for my body. Instead, I doubled down and became even harder-core and more aggressive about a vegan lifestyle.

Then, in early 2018, I was diagnosed with prediabetes.

(Record scratch) Wait–what? How can someone who weighs under 100 lbs. (45kg) and who doesn't eat sweets be prediabetic? That's not a thing, is it?

How in the world did I get here?

Well, I was steeped in an ego-driven world that said my worth as a woman was strongly correlated with how skinny and hot (aka fuckable) I looked. It said I was never meant to look older than 25. And it cared only about my outward appearance.

And I had believed it.

Instead of listening to my body as it gently whispered to me, then spoke a little more urgently, and now was screaming at me, I got annoyed with it, ignored its urgent attempts to communicate, and prioritized external pressure rather than internal *knowing*.

Then, while I was at the gym (again), sweating profusely on the treadmill (again) as I sought to work off all the fat I had eaten (again), fearful it would make me gain weight (again), I started watching a podcast with that same Dave Asprey guy, and he was talking about biohacking again with his guest.

I was even more intrigued—and desperate—so I started reading up more on the whole concept. That was when I learned about some of the "O.G." biohackers like Dr. Weston Price and the philosophies they espouse.

Once I started implementing the techniques I am about to share with you in this book, I couldn't believe the changes in my body and mind! I felt strong. I felt at home inside my body. I felt like I was finally able to think of something other than my body and food alone.

I also felt like I had lost precious years of my life by focusing on diets and misinformation instead of growing as a human being and using all that energy for something else, like learning an instrument, dancing, or becoming better at skydiving (which is my passion).

This was the start of everything changing both within me and for me. My body was already waving its hands up and down in the air, flashing neon signs at me; all I had to do was listen, learn, and pivot.

But that can be the most difficult and confusing part. We live in an age of SO MUCH information that it opens the door to the risk of misinformation, too. And even if the information accessible to us is fine and accurate, how do we piece it all together? How do we put it into practice? How do we know what will work for our bodies without wasting years trying to implement plans that work for other people but don't—and possibly never will—align with our unique biology?

I know what it's like to feel like your physique doesn't match your mentality and energy for life. Feeling like your body isn't "listening" to you is a terrible feeling. But what if I told you that I learned to flip that on its head and ask myself, "What if it's *me* who's not listening to *my body* and what it's been trying to tell me?"

My mission is to help women rebuild their relationship with food. My goal is to get you so proficient at reading your body that you don't look at diets thinking, "Maybe this will work." You will be so fluent in yourself that you will only have one diet, and that diet is called: I DO WHAT WORKS FOR ME.

There is no such thing as "one size fits all." This is why you will often hear me—and anyone within the health industry who truly cares—insist that *diets don't work*. Lifestyle does. Biohacking is not a diet. It's a lifestyle.

Okay. So, by this point, I'm sure you're ready to roll, and so am I. I just want to ensure we are clear on a few more things before we jump into this together.

Manifesto of a Biohacker

There are some truths you need to believe about yourself, and I'm going to ask you to read through this list—aloud if you can. (I mean, if you're reading this on public transportation, you might garner some weird looks. But hey, that's okay, too!) Take a deep breath, and repeat after me:

I am a heroine—a true main character in the movie called *My Wonderful Life*.

I know the essence of who I truly am—radiance, joy, love—and my mission is to embody these qualities every day.

I take accountability and extreme ownership for my choices and actions. I choose to speak only words of empowerment. "I have to" or "I can't" are phrases that do not exist in my vocabulary.

I understand that taking care of myself is not a selfish luxury but my top priority. I am always hungry for knowledge, for asking questions, and for seeking to understand how everything in my environment affects my health, my energy, and my aura.

I never shy away from speaking out loud or taking up space. My presence commands attention; warmth radiates from within me. My greatest joy comes from lifting other queens up alongside me.

As a biohacker, I'm relentless in pursuing physical and mental well-being. I know that the best biohacks come from cutting-edge technology and from nature—practices like basking in the sun, practicing meditation, connecting with the community, and mastering breathwork.

My legacy is built on love, healing, and breaking the cycle. Symptoms do not define me; they are merely feedback from my body. And so, I continue to explore new techniques and experiment with biohacking to optimize my health and well-being.

Unprocessed emotions and experiences are stored as trauma in the body, but fear or self-doubt will never hold me back. Instead, I embody power and confidence fit for a queen.

As a biohacker, I don't need anyone's approval or permission. I own every aspect of who I am without apology or hesitation. Nothing can tame this woman; she stands tall like a beacon of light, illuminating even the darkest corners of the world around us.

Focus on What You Already Are

I once read, "You can't build on top of success you haven't acknowledged." So before we go any further and before I bombard you with all the biohacking secrets, let's acknowledge you and everything you have been and are already doing.

I'll start: You're curious. And you're smart (I mean, you just picked up a book on science and biology. Come on—that's got to count for something!). You are connected with your intuition. Deep down in your soul, you feel that struggling is not where you belong, and the mainstream fitness advice doesn't resonate with you and doesn't leave your body feeling like its best self for the long term.

Now, let's write down all the things you are already doing (you are probably already biohacking and just don't know it!). Maybe it's daily walking or that healthy salad you picked over pizza the other day. Or maybe you had pizza, which made you feel good because you needed comfort food then. Good job! You are listening to your body!

It's so easy to focus on the lack, on the negative, or on seeking unattainable versions of our body and lifestyle. That is our Perfect Self in action. I'll explain a little bit more about her later, but for now, let's just say that she's the mean stepsister living in your head, saying, "Ugh, look at that cellulite" or "I look fat" every time she sees herself in the photo. Or the one who constantly berates you for not doing a diet right. Or the one who feels like she always needs to implement ALL THE BIOHACKS ALL THE TIME.

Perfect Self is feeding us the idea that if we look perfect (shed unrealistic amounts of weight, grow thick hair like we're in a shampoo commercial, clear out our skin like some ridiculous photo filter), our life will get better. The truth is: It won't. Skinny people hate themselves, too. People with flawless hair and skin have miserable lives, too.

I don't want you to biohack from a place of desperation and aspiration but from a place of curiosity. I mean, sure, you've got goals. Of course you do, and that's wonderful and powerful and good. But the truth is, your body is performing millions of mini-tasks every second, and 99% of them are performed so seamlessly you don't even notice. Our primary focus is to support her and see how much better she might feel if we gave her some loving assistance as she does her job day in, day out.

And because we are curious about how to best support our bodies, it's important to ask yourself a couple of questions: Why am I here? What made me pick up this book? Am I here because I don't want to look a certain way? Am I here because I feel resentful toward my body, and why it's *not listening to me?* Am I here because I want to know why my body is not looking like the body of a supermodel?

The energy behind every decision you make changes the outcome. I'm not going to lie; the first time I got into biohacking, the primary question in my head I was trying to find the answer to was: "What is wrong with me and my annoying body, and how can I fix it?" Spoiler alert: I needed to fix my mindset, not my body.

Today, I understand that it was *not my body not listening* to me, it was *me* not listening to my body. All she wanted was for me to stop following fad diets full of sugar, snacking, and drinking so many smoothies that I almost forgot how to chew. She wanted me to stop thinking about what I should be eating all the time and start *living*.

I want you to know it's okay if you're here for the same reason. But I'd love to invite you to add a couple of new reasons. You know, just for fun.

Instead of:

- I want to lose belly fat.
- I want to stop being sick.
- I want to shed some unwanted weight.
- I want to find out what's wrong with my skin/ my hormones/ me.
- I am here to follow all the rules, like I'm back in school so I can be a good girl and get an A+.

Let's try:

- I want to feel good in my body more often.
- I am here to let my body heal herself.
- I'm here to rebuild the relationship with my body.
- I want to learn to listen to what my body says.
- I'm here to understand science and do what feels right and best for myself and my body.
- I'm here to love myself more than ever before.
- I'm here to feel light and strong and at home in my body.
- Screw being a good girl and getting things perfect. I do my best as I go, but I aim for growth, not perfection.

So if you're constantly worried about your stomach being bloated and most of your thought energy seems to be focused around,

"What do I do about my bloated stomach? I don't want to feel this way. I want to get rid of the love handles and cellulite."

What if you tried this instead? "I love my hands; they are beautiful. I love how I use them every day: washing my face, typing on my phone or laptop, meeting new people, or cooking delicious meals. They never complain, they are never tired, they never take a day off. They always help me accomplish my goals, whether they're as small as squeezing a lemon in the morning or as big as doing my job each day. I am so sorry I never praised you guys. Each finger separately or as a collective. I love you. I adore you. I appreciate you."

Did loving your body for a minute rather than criticizing it feel good? Let's keep going!

"I absolutely love my knees. Gosh, aren't they incredibly reliable? I squat, I walk, I sit, and they are always there for me. I wouldn't go places, see my friends, or travel the world if it wasn't for you guys. You look kind of funny, like a shar-pei puppy's face, but who doesn't love a puppy? You are incredible."

"My teeth. I have never praised each of you separately, especially those in the back, doing all the hard work of chewing. Thank you for letting me enjoy delicious food. I love you."

"And speaking of eating, my tongue and my dear taste buds, I freaking love you, too. Each one of you: the sour, the sweet, the bitter, the salty, the umami. I have built my life around you (though maybe sometimes I over-rely on the sweet guys and let the bitter ones get a little bored), yet I never really stop to say thank you. I appreciate you. I get to speak thanks to this incredible muscle that my tongue is. I love the fact I get to speak and communicate with my soul, and I love my voice."

This exercise could go on forever. You can love your heart for never taking a day off. You can love your eyes for letting you read fun books, your ears for listening to your favorite music, your lungs for drawing in and exhaling air, and your liver for detoxifying you after a night out ...

Your Higher Self understands that she's here to appreciate and love everything that her body is already doing and to learn how she can support it with the right diet to make it easier for the parts that are overworked and struggling to work on an optimal level. Take a moment to acknowledge how incredible that really is—how incredible *you* really are.

You are not here to play small. You are not here to just get by. You are here not just to survive but to thrive.

You are here to unleash your superpowers, step into your main character energy, and be the queen of your destiny.

Your lower self may have been running the show up to now, but the truth is, you can put your Higher Self in charge of the rest of your life. The ultimate goal of this book is to help you consistently access your Higher Self.

Now, with an open heart chakra, fuzzy from all the gratitude and appreciation toward our incredible bodies, let's dive in.

Love Your Fat

When I launched my first biohacking course, I welcomed over 1,500 women who had never heard of biohacking but were very familiar with dieting, counting calories, and being hard on themselves and their bodies. One of the first videos I released was called "Love Your Fat" because I knew that this perspective shift was essential for everything else to make sense.

In this video, I say, "If you are here, chances are you have been try-ing to lose fat for a good portion of your life. You have probably looked in the mirror or at a photo of yourself and rolled your eyes, thinking, *Oh, I look fat,* or *I hate my fat.* You've probably googled 'how to lose belly fat' or 'how to lose weight' at least once in your life."

But let's be honest: you don't have to google or look for diet informa-tion to hear the unsolicited advice. It's everywhere. We live in a diet culture. You and I are bombarded with advice that goes along the lines of "Come on, what's wrong with you? Just eat less, move your bum more, and you'll be fit."

We are considered lazy if we don't have the energy to work out.

Broken if we can't lose weight.

Not motivated enough when we eat something unhealthy.

Looked down upon because we are lost in the sea of (mis)information.

It only takes about five seconds on social media to believe something is wrong with us for not already doing something that someone believes is the only correct way to live. Wait, you don't do Pilates? Wait, you don't drink this drink when you wake up? Omg, you don't X, Y, and Z? No wonder you're struggling. *It's your own damn fault.*

The diet culture perpetuates and repeats what you already tell your-self in your head: *I am not good enough, skinny enough, and motivated/ smart/sexy enough.*

I was doing a morning meditation in Bali right after the "Love Your Fat" video dropped, and that was when the idea for this book came to me. We had just started to hear from people who were blown away by the revelation of an idea as simple as embracing their fat, and I knew that the message needed to go bigger than just that audi-ence of 1,500 people. This book was born from a place of serenity and beauty, and I think that is so apt because it's meant to take you from frustration and overwhelm to overwhelming peace and joy.

If you only knew what your fat does for you, you would never look in the mirror and hate it again! Let's take a moment to clear the air between you and your fat cells.

Have you ever paused and deeply contemplated how you feel within the contours of your body? It's not just about the tangible sense of touch or comfort, but an emotional and psychological alignment—or, sometimes, a profound lack thereof.

For some, the body serves as a haven, a familiar refuge. But for others (maybe you), it may feel more like an unfamiliar or even hostile terrain.

When you look in the mirror, what do you *feel*? Do you get overwhelmed with feelings of estrangement or unease? It's fascinating how our internal perception of our external "human suit" can cast long shadows over our interactions, self-esteem, and even our mental well-being. Not feeling safe or connected to your body can be a heavy thing to carry, affecting not just your relationship with yourself but also with the world at large. Such feelings may beckon a deeper understanding and perhaps a journey toward reconciliation with yourself.

Let's start by reconciling with those fat cells.

Have you ever wondered what fat cells do? No, they don't only make you "look fat."

I like to think of my fat as my "safety suit." We store fat for two main reasons. First, it's there to protect our organs like a thermal insulator and bubble wrap combined. Secondly, fat releases hormones like leptin, which regulates appetite and energy and stores fat-soluble hormones, such as vitamin D. Thirdly, just like a good house husband, the body likes to have a secret stash of food (nutrients) for a rainy day. Fat is a storage for energy to pull from whenever there is a caloric deficit, such as during fasting or intense physical activity.

Now, if you have some extra fat, it's likely your body is overwhelmed with all the processes she's already doing. She's either getting too many toxins, which confuse her hormones, or too much sugar that she can't metabolize fast enough. So, to make sure you don't die, she stashes that sugar in your fat cells in case she needs it later. That means that fat is actually *protecting* you from a challenging lifestyle and diet circumstances.

Here's the thing: When your body does not feel safe, and your sympathetic nervous system (the part of your brain that regulates the flight-flight-freeze-fawn response) is in high gear, there is a message circulating to every organ, tissue, and cell of your body, sounding the alarm: "What's happening out there is very unpredictable." The automatic parts of your brain-body connection can't distinguish between stress caused by a deadline at work and stress caused by the possibility of having to hide in the forest from a tiger for a week with very little food. All it knows is that its primary job is to keep you alive, so it will start stashing away some extra fat to ensure you have provisions for survival.

You'll hear me say over and over in the book: fasting without feasting is starvation, and pushing your body without appropriate rest is torture. Mainstream starvation diets put our bodies in a constant state of stress: intense workouts lead to calorie deficits when paired with a strict, low-fat diet. The body can't grasp that this is deliberate and intentional stress; all it knows is it is time to go into safety mode.

When my grandma died, my mom put on 20 kg in three months, and it wasn't only emotional eating. My grandmother was a single mother, raising my mom solo in Cold War-era Poland. She was my mom's primary sense of safety in this world, so when she died, my mom felt like her entire world collapsed; hence, she put on 20 kilos of "safety suit."

A lot of what I do with my students and practice on my own with my spiritual coach is to restore the sense of safety in our bodies and in the world.

At this point in my life, my sense of safety is just being present with what comes up. But this wasn't always the case. I used to go out of my way to avoid uncomfortable feelings, especially fear.

When I started skydiving, however, I decided to take a different approach. There was nowhere to hide from my fear, even though it was making me dizzy and sick to my stomach. I know that my fear is always a combination of:

1. what's in front of me, and
2. all the unfaced fears I have been avoiding for years: fear of getting old, fear of missing out, fear of abandonment.

I also know that it's okay to sit with it. To acknowledge it. It's okay to be scared and overwhelmed. Do you believe that for yourself? I hope so.

Let's have a little heart-to-heart about our bodies. First off, name three things about yours that you're genuinely thankful for today. Got 'em? Awesome. Now, think about that moment when you're super comfy in your skin. Maybe it's chilling on your couch or laughing with friends. What about those times when you feel like an absolute boss—like when you're dancing, hiking, pursuing a hobby that gives you life, or just doing everyday stuff? Now, here's a deeper one: What does it feel like to truly feel safe in your body? Can you remember when your body totally wowed you with its strength or bounce-back game?

Let's talk about the simple things, like how amazing the feeling of warm sun is on your skin or the comforting sensation of a cozy blanket. Have you ever noticed how great it feels to take a deep, nourishing breath? And what about those moments when you get a strong gut feeling or a sudden burst of energy like your body's trying to tell you something? Think about those things. Think about everything your body can do and everything it has already done. How can you honor its constant efforts to keep you safe? How can you trust it, even through your fear? How can you acknowledge that its automatic responses (which you may not always love) are evidence of the hard work of keeping you alive? How can you be 100% present in your body—fat cells and all—even for just a moment or two today?

Make Friends With Your Fat

Here are some journal prompts to help you embrace and love your body fat:

1. List three ways your body fat has served you in the past. This could include providing energy, keeping you warm, or protecting your organs.
2. Write a letter to your body fat, thanking it for the ways it supports your health and well-being. Now write another letter apologizing to your fat cells for all the times you hated them.
3. Write a letter to your future self and thank it for the many things it will see you through and protect you in the coming weeks, months, and years.
4. How does your body feel when you embrace all parts of it, including your fat? How does it feel to know that you are perfect the way you are, and there's nothing you need to do to become healthier, prettier, or better? Describe these sensations.

5. Body fat is a superpower because it helps us survive and thrive. How does it feel to think about your body fat in this way?

6. Think about the warmth provided by body fat in cold weather. How does this make you feel about your body fat?

Remember, every part of your body, including your body fat, contributes to the unique, beautiful individual that you are. It's more than okay to appreciate and love all aspects of your body.

Here is my letter to my fat cells:

Dear Fat Cells,

I want to apologize to you. I now realize that for far too long, I've looked at you through a lens of criticism, resentment, and even hatred. I've failed to see you for what you truly are—a vital part of me, essential for my survival, well-being, and strength.

I'm sorry for the times I stood in front of the mirror and wished you away, not appreciating your importance. I've misunderstood your role, not recognizing that you are a part of my body's intricate and beautifully complex system designed to protect and nourish me.

I have unfairly labeled you as unwanted, undesirable, and a symbol of imperfection. I now realize that you are an integral part of me, working tirelessly to protect and support my well-being.

You store energy for me, helping me get through long days, intense workouts, and periods of illness. You help keep me warm, protect my organs, and even have a role in producing hormones that regulate important bodily functions.

In my ignorance, I've blamed you for societal standards that are often unrealistic and unhealthy, not understanding that you are not a reflection of my worth. I've allowed external voices and influences to dictate how I feel about you, forgetting that your purpose goes far beyond aesthetics.

I apologize for succumbing to societal pressures and unrealistic beauty standards that demanded you be anything other than what you are. I have compared you to others, believing that you define my worth when, in reality, your presence has nothing to do with my value as a person.

You have been there for me through thick and thin (literally!), providing insulation, cushioning, and energy storage when needed. You have acted as a faithful guardian, preventing harm and regulating various bodily processes. Your existence has allowed me to survive and thrive. For that, I am genuinely thankful.

I regret all the times I subjected you to extreme diets, harmful habits, and unattainable expectations. I pushed you to the limits, expecting you to fit into an unrealistic mold that goes against your natural purpose. I now understand that this was not only unfair but harmful to our relationship.

From this moment forward, I promise to embrace you with love and compassion.

Instead of focusing on how you make me look, I will appreciate how you contribute to my health and survival.

I will work on loving you, as part of loving myself.

I'm sorry for the times I've failed to see your value.

Thank you for your continued service to my body, even when I didn't appreciate it. I am grateful for you. I love you. I love doing life with you.

With all my love and gratitude,

—Aggie

Why You Are Struggling

In the movie *Good Will Hunting*, Matt Damon's character (Will) had a tough childhood and was constantly in trouble. When his therapist, played by Robin Williams, says to him, "It's not your fault," Will dismisses it at first and says, "Yeah, okay, I know. It's not my fault."

But then they go back and forth a few times, and for almost a full minute, his therapist says it over and over again: "It's not your fault. It's not your fault. It's not your fault." Will finally breaks down when the message sinks in. And that is my message to you. It's not your fault. Please let that sink in.

It's not your fault.

Things like PMS, hormonal acne, unexpected weight gain or weight loss, intense cravings, mood swings and irritability, brittle or thinning hair, premature wrinkles, energy crashes, bloating, water retention, painful or irregular periods, heavy periods, anxiety, overwhelm, depression, feeling broken, not wanting to leave the house—these are all *common*, but they're not *normal*.

They're all signs of dysregulated hormones. And they aren't your fault.

When I was struggling with severe acne, I went to the dermatologist and ended up going on the strongest medication available at the time. This stuff is so damaging that you have to sign a waiver saying you'll use two forms of birth control if you're sexually active.

I was on it not once, but twice. If I knew then what I know now, I would have looked at that as a prescription for ruining my liver, triggering depression, and preventing me from fixing my diet so I could actually find the root cause of my acne.

As women, we are exposed to approximately 168 different chemicals (about twice as many as men) per day. *Per day!* No one knows the long-term effects of all of these chemicals, but we do know that high toxin levels and diets low in nutrients lead to infertility and hormonal issues.

If you feel out of sync with your body, there's a root cause.

If you've tried everything, but nothing seems to work, the problem isn't your lack of effort.

If you've ever tried to lose weight and failed, it's not because you're lazy or you're not eating less and running more.

If your sex drive is suffering, you're not alone.

If your mood swings are so intense that they're interfering with your relationships or risking your job, there's a reason for that.

If it feels like your hormones are controlling you, they are.

What if the solution to these problems was as simple as regulating your hormones? Would a few changes be worth it?

If you're willing to make positive, lasting changes to your lifestyle to balance your hormones naturally but don't know where to start, you're in the right place.

This quickstart guide will help you sift through all of the conflicting information about hormonal health (much of which is either targeted toward men or backed by the self-serving pharmaceutical industry) and help you get back to feeling energetic, confident, fit, and healthy again.

You deserve to wake up without dark circles under your eyes.

You deserve to have so much energy that you jump out of bed feeling rested and refreshed without needing coffee to start your day.

You deserve to have clear, beautiful skin.

You deserve to have a body that you feel great in.

You deserve to feel energized.

Today is Day 1 of your journey.

My friend Jim Kwik says: "The first time, it's a mistake; the second time, it's a choice." Now that you have this book in your hands, make sure you don't choose the struggle again.

Say Goodbye to Starvation Diets

As I mentioned earlier, my family called me "Little Dumpling" growing up. As time went on, I took on the identity of being chubby. I acted like a dumpling. My body acted like a dumpling.

Then, when I was about 25 years old, I decided to start working out at a gym and finally shed that identity. I felt weak, out of place, awkward, lost, and stared at. I had no idea what I was doing. Being chubby and out of place at the gym was my identity now.

I wanted to still look like me—to still look like a woman and radiate feminine energy—but to be a more flexible and stronger version of myself.

Eventually, I realized that all these identities I was taking on— Dumpling, Gym Newbie—weren't serving me, so I decided to take on the identity of an athlete. Because ... well, why the hell not?

Then I started living from that place.

I wouldn't just work out, I trained. (That's what athletes do, right?) I pushed myself until the sweat was dripping down my forehead because that's what I saw athletes do in the movies. I wasn't changing my goals, just the mindset behind my goals.

This was one of my first forays into biohacking, even though I had no idea about it at the time. It's about changing our mindset to embrace a different way of inhabiting our space—a way of life that includes breathwork, discipline, gratitude, fitness/training, and learning how to understand the environment we live in so we can set ourselves up for success.

People were designed with an integral sense of intuition that has been our body's way of speaking to us, telling us what's right and wrong for us, good and bad, threatening or nurturing, for hundreds of thousands of years of human evolution.

But then we started outsourcing our power to "experts" instead of relying on that intuition. Biohacking allows us to take back that power by listening to science and then asking ourselves, "Which parts of the science work *for me*, where I am right now, and how can I apply them? There is no linear or fast path to success, mastery, or fitness. It's a continuous, lifelong commitment to listening to your body and adapting—just as you were designed to do.

And those adaptations need to start with your mindset around food.

You're a Biohacker, Not a Dieter

An older monk and a younger monk were traveling and came upon a river with a strong current. As they were about to cross, they noticed a young woman who also wanted to cross but was having trouble. She asked them for help. The monks, who had taken vows not to touch women, exchanged a look. Then, without saying anything, the senior monk picked her up, carried her across the river, and set her down gently on the other side before continuing their journey.

The younger monk couldn't believe what he just saw. He rejoined his companion but did not speak for a full hour.

Two more hours passed without a word between them, then three. Finally, the younger monk could no longer contain himself. "As monks, we are not permitted to touch a woman. Why did you dare to carry the woman on your shoulders?"

The older monk looked at him and gently replied, "Brother, I set her down on the other side of the river. Why are you still carrying her?"

The dieting mindset is a bit like that junior monk. You carry around all the "right" things you are supposed to eat and the list of dos and don'ts in your head. It's impossible to put them down, and they eventually become the only thing on your mind.

I used to go to birthday parties and circle the kitchen the entire time, nibbling on anything my hand could reach way before everyone else was interested in looking at the food.

I looked at all the fit people in the room chatting and having fun and not obsessing (yes, that's the right word) about when the food was going to be served. They didn't overeat as I did, and they also had all the carbs and dessert without any guilt. They ate when it was time and enjoyed the party. Meanwhile, I was the one nibbling beforehand, reactively restricting myself during the meal, and then feeling guilty afterward for not being like other people and having one guilt-free cookie or a single scoop of ice cream without it turning into a Whole Thing.

A big part of my identity shift from calorie-restricted dieting to biohacking is that I moved from trying to remain in a constant calorie deficit to consuming more calories than the so-called daily recommendations.

The whole concept of using calorie restriction to lose weight is based on a flawed premise that your basal metabolic rate (BMR) always stays the same, so if you consume less than that, you will lose weight. And you will, in the short term, but your basal metabolic rate will shortly adjust to operate on an even smaller amount of calories, and you will then have to eat even less to keep losing weight.

For example, if my BMR is 1,500 calories and I only eat 1,400 calories, I will lose weight. But before too long, my body will adjust my basal metabolic rate to 1,300 calories because it's intelligent and wants to keep storing fat to keep me alive. Meanwhile, if I am still consuming 1,400 calories, I will hit a plateau and then yo-yo back to my original weight, if not higher.

Metabolic Compensation

Your body doesn't care about fitting into a new pair of jeans. Her job is to keep you alive. One way she does that is by using something called "metabolic compensation." It's your body's sneaky way of resisting change when you're trying to lose weight.

Let's say you decide to shed some weight by cutting your calorie intake or increasing your physical activity (aka almost every diet in the world). You start to lose weight. You're thrilled. You think, "Finally! Something that works!"

But then your body hits the "panic" button. It doesn't like change, and it's especially protective of its fat reserves (an evolutionary trick to survive famines, you will recall). A continuous food shortage sends one message to the brain: *Girl, things are changing out there! Food is getting more and more scarce!*

Remember, your body's job is to ensure you have enough energy for survival. It doesn't care how you look on the beach in a two-piece swimsuit. When you consistently give your body too few calories, it adjusts by slowing down processes and becoming more efficient in utilizing the fuel you provide.

In other words, your body starts to adjust your metabolism by becoming super efficient at using fewer calories to perform the same tasks. It's like your body switches from an old diesel truck to a fuel-efficient Tesla. And guess what else? Your body will also start sending stronger hunger signals, making you want to eat more.

This is the metabolic compensation kicking in, making weight loss a moving target and often contributing to the dreaded "yo-yo effect" of dieting, where people lose weight only to regain it when the diet ends.

However, it's not all doom and gloom. Understanding metabolic compensation can help you make sustainable lifestyle changes rather than relying on quick fixes. Small, gradual changes in eating habits and regular physical activity that includes strength training can help overcome the body's resistance to weight loss.

While metabolic compensation might seem annoying, it's just your body trying to look out for you. But with the right strategies, you can coax it into embracing the new, healthier you.

The way you eat is not supposed to make you feel miserable. But when something feels good, we often think, *Oh, that can't be healthy. This probably isn't going to work.*

The good news is the opposite is true.

Say Hello to Biohacking Levels

I am about to share with you the Biohacking Eating Lifestyle™, but if you are new to biohacking, stick to Level 1 for at least a month. In fact, no matter where you are on this journey, please don't start with any drastic changes to your diet.

Why? Well, for starters, I want to see you win. And you will, no question about it.

But if your diet is poor, drastically removing every speck of sugar when your entire biology is screaming, "Give me the donut!" is going to make you absolutely miserable. You will end up throwing darts into a picture of me and calling biohacking "torture," "cruel and unusual punishment," or "truly the worst idea ever, and why did I ever think this was anything I could do and I hate it, and I hate Aggie, and I hate everything, and I still don't have that damn donut."

We're not here to suffer and struggle. We're here to hack your biology so that eating healthy feels fun and painless. Because it's meant to be. If it's not, it's not biohacking. We're not obsessing, not restricting, and definitely not limiting ourselves to small portions. It's a way to navigate the reality of the food landscape these days.

We have our preferences (some are stronger than others), but at the end of the day, I want you to feel expansive and free while still bringing about the results you dream of—whether it's deflating your fat cells, getting more energy, or improving your sex drive.

We're not transforming you into someone else. We're helping you return to your fullest expression, the most energetic, playful version of yourself. That's your birthright: to feel freaking incredible in your own body and not settle for anything less.

4 Levels of Becoming a Biohacker

Becoming an independent biohacker is similar to progressing through the iconic world of a Super Mario game on PlayStation. I used to love playing that with my sister, and while this won't involve throwing turtle shells at your enemies (please be nice to turtles!), it will definitely make you feel like you are moving at turbo speed with incredible strength. (Or something like that. Did I take the metaphor too far? Yes? No? Are you rolling your eyes right now? Well, brace yourself because things are about to get even more Mario-y.)

Level 1: The When/Timing

In Level 1 of your biohacking journey, you're hanging out in the Mushroom Kingdom (Anyone? Please?) You're not matching your diet to your genetic makeup or trying photobiomodulation or rectal ozone administration—or even trying to pronounce them. You'll get there—both trying and pronouncing them—but they are nothing to focus on right now. This level is about the basics.

All you're doing right now is strategically altering the timing and sequence of your current diet to work in harmony with your body's natural rhythms. Just a few smart tweaks. No drastic changes. No spending money on gadgets, weird grocery items, or fancy testing. You will not have to spend a single dollar more (actually, you will probably *save* money) at this level.

Here's how you do it: You eat your food in the right order, condense everything you eat into three meals a day, and limit your eating window.

And … that's it.

What? That's it?!?! Aggie, that can't be! Surely there's a catch.

Nope. At Level 1, that's all you need to worry about. These shifts might seem small, but these timing adjustments of your food will improve your hormones, help you feel less hangry (you know what you're like), give you fewer cravings, and help you lose a few pounds while you're at it.

Level 2: What and What Not to Eat

Now you've smashed a few blocks, discovered the fire flower (you knew that was coming), and you're ready to level up. After a few weeks of having your biology adjusted, it's gonna leave you hungry (pun intended) for more. Your glucose will be regulated, and your hunger hormones will be in much better shape. You'll feel lighter, better, less bloated, and will crave better food. You'll be hungry for more. Then, and only then, can you start implementing the suggestions below. If, at any point in your biohacking journey, you notice yourself feeling overwhelmed, go back to Level 1 and stay there as long as you need. The world doesn't need another hard-core biohacker; it needs you to be happy and not overwhelmed.

We'll get into the details of Level 2 below, thinking about how to navigate a grocery store to pick food that will nourish you instead of making you sick. We'll also chat about things most biohackers avoid to help protect and increase our energy to stay healthy and fit.

Level 3: Embrace Your Cycle

Once you've passed Levels 1 and 2, you'll be bursting with energy. You're Mario grabbing the Starman. In Level 3, you'll become a pro at living according to your menstrual cycle; you'll know when and how to train, when to rest, and when to push yourself. Did you know that if you overtrain yourself at the wrong part of your cycle, you can actually gain weight instead of losing it? *Like—what? Why did no one tell us this in 5th grade?*

Level 4: Live Like a Biohacker

You are now an advanced biohacker, and just as Mario can grab the Super Leaf to gain the ears and tail of a raccoon, giving him the ability to fly (though raccoons can't actually fly, so that feels a bit weird?), you will be soaring to new heights. You'll want to become really good in bed (*I'm* talking about sleep. What were *you* thinking?), combat stress, and create an environment that will support your energy. Again, I made sure that everything I recommend in the book will not cost you an arm or a leg—or a raccoon tail.

Each level in biohacking, just like in Super Mario, builds on the last, offering new challenges and opportunities for growth. You start by mastering the basics and progress to a point where you're not just playing the game, you're setting new high scores in your personal health and well-being.

Bio-Slacker 20% of the Time

Now, I have a disclaimer—just a little caveat. (Okay, actually, it's a really big one.)

As you grow into your biohacker identity, you need to adopt a second and equally important identity: that of a bio-slacker—20% of the time. Yep, you heard that right. You are going to be an epic biohacker 80% of the time, and the other 20% of the time, you're just gonna get it wrong, break the rules, and completely f*ck up everything you learn.

Why? Because I don't want you to make the mistake I did when I first became a vegan and then made again when I first became a biohacker. I was so worried and obsessed about what to eat and what not to eat I would spend 20 minutes reading the menu at every restaurant, obsessing about every ingredient. I was tense, stressed, and kept worrying about every meal. There is a term for it now: it's called *orthorexia*, which is an unhealthy focus on eating in a healthy way.

I'M GOING TO KEEP REPEATING IT OVER AND OVER AGAIN: Too much of a good thing is bad. My Fit as F*ck students used to message me all the time: "Aggie, what do I do? I can't live without tomatoes/oat milk/coffee/donuts/chocolate/etc."

And I would respond, "So don't. Do everything else. Get all the other things right and include the donuts in the 20%."

This approach is not only more doable, more human, and more fun, but it's also more realistic for someone living in the 21st century.

People will ask me, "How can you paint your nails, buy drugstore makeup, or use products in your hair? I thought you were a biohacker?!" While I understand super hard-core biohackers get so many things right, getting everything "right" is no longer my goal. I also don't plan to live until I'm 180. What I want is to get the most out of the years I've got. I'll bet you do, too.

"Aggie!!! After doing your Fit as F*ck course, I started making small changes to my diet, mainly level 1 hacks. I don't know how much weight I lost because I don't own a scale—but after less than a month, I look better than I did when I was 18 years old, and I finally have the energy to run after my 'two under two'! And the best part? For the first time in over 20 years, I don't feel like I am on a diet. It's the most freeing feeling! Thank you a million times, thank you!!!"

—Martha, 39

KEY TAKEAWAYS

- Embrace biohacking as a lifestyle, focusing on listening to your body and making informed, personalized health choices rather than adhering to restrictive, one-size-fits-all diets.

- Understand that struggles with weight, mood swings, and other health issues are often rooted in hormonal imbalances and external factors, not personal failings.

- Recognize the importance of self-love and appreciation for your body, including aspects like body fat, as they play crucial roles in your overall health and well-being.

- Adopt a mindset shift from viewing yourself as a chronic dieter to being a biohacker, prioritizing intuitive eating and lifestyle changes over calorie counting.

- Implement gradual, sustainable changes in your diet and lifestyle, respecting your body's natural rhythms and needs and allowing room for flexibility and self-compassion.

LEVEL 1:
WHEN TO EAT

CHAPTER 2

EAT IN THE RIGHT ORDER

Y ou will start your biohacking journey with … changing *nothing* about your diet. Yep, that's right. Nothing. Nada. Nichts. Continue eating as you normally would, without stressing whether it's biohacking-approved or not. The only difference? Eat your food in the right order and at the right time of the day.

Why? Because science proves that you and I can have the exact same diet and the same amount of calories, yet I'll lose weight and you'll gain or vice versa. You'll think something is wrong with you, but there isn't. You just weren't biohacking.

Here is the kicker: You can continue with the same diet and the same food but change the order you eat it in and change the timing of it throughout the day, and chances are you'll be looking at more regulated hormones, more energy, and even better skin.

If you currently have five meals a day, start your day with a sweet breakfast or a latte, and love to start each meal with a dinner roll, please read on. The next few pages are going to be a game changer.

Here are your first three steps:

- **Eat your food in the right order:** Become more mindful of the order in which you consume foods within a meal. Starting with fiber-rich vegetables and proteins can lead to a more gradual rise in blood glucose levels, rather than spiking them with simple carbs right off the bat.

- **Condense everything you eat to three meals a day:** Instead of grazing throughout the day on nuts, lattes, or hummus with carrots, these "microfasts" allow your digestive system to rest and reset, much like Mario finding a moment of respite in a safe castle before heading back into the fray.

- **Limit your "eating window":** Set your meal time between breakfast and dinner—roughly a 12-hour span—and commit to that. Perhaps start with breakfast at 7 a.m. and finish dinner by 7 p.m., aligning with natural daylight hours to support your metabolism. Look at that—you're already doing intermittent fasting! Eventually, we will want to work your way up to fasting for 14, 15, and even 16 hours (at the right time of your cycle), but starting small is important.

And … that's it.

But let's take a deeper dive into these steps because I want you to understand what's really going on with your body and how these steps contribute to creating your healthiest and most radiant life.

Glucose: Have Your Cake and Eat It

Imagine a world where you can have your favorite dish without racking up all the guilt and gut pain that inevitably comes with it. The phrase "You can't have your cake and eat it too" has come to mean that we need to prioritize our desires and make choices accordingly.

But why would you want to have cake ... and *not* eat it? Would it just be for looking at? Where's the fun in that?

The thing is, it *is* possible to enjoy the short-term pleasure of a sweet treat or pizza while not paying the price for it with your health and fitness goals! That's right: I'm talking about *literally* having your cake *and eating* it. Too good to be true? It's not! It's all about understanding the science behind glucose and using it to your advantage and pleasure—because life is too short not to have that croissant!

Remember when I said I started "dieting" when I was 12 years old? I knew that "Dumpling" wasn't cute for a teenage girl, and I feared eating full meals. I eventually swapped out my mother's egg and sausage breakfasts for something I thought was lighter because I decided that eating meat would make me even fatter. (I wasn't too far off as industrial and processed meats are awful, but more on that later). I decided instead to start having cereal for breakfast—usually anything labeled as "fitness," which often meant that the pieces were coated with "yogurt" (basically just a combination of high fructose corn syrup and condensed milk).

For lunch, I had a latte with juice because "proper food" felt scary. Again, more sugar. I was starting and continuing my day with a high amount of pure sugar, which meant I was living in a series of massive glucose spikes, although I had no idea at the time what that even was and just how badly it would screw up my hormones.

Then, I had my vegan phase after I moved to LA. I had always assumed that skinny equals healthy (wrong!), so I was shocked when I started struggling. I couldn't go more than two hours without feeling hungry and weak, and it seemed like most of my time was spent thinking about my next meal.

The thing is, sugar levels matter not only because of potential diabetes but because sugar ages us, screws up our hormones and fertility, leads to acne and hair loss, impacts our energy, and makes us moody. And yet, we can't seem to stop consuming it.

In 2019, I started wearing a continuous glucose monitor (CGM), a device that keeps track of blood sugar levels throughout the day to help me understand what food impacts my sugar in real time. Here's what I learned.

Oat milk latte first thing in the morning: up 50.

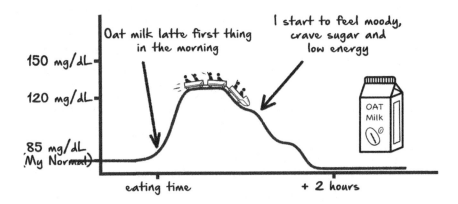

Oat milk latte first thing in the morning in a to-go cup followed by a walk: up 25.

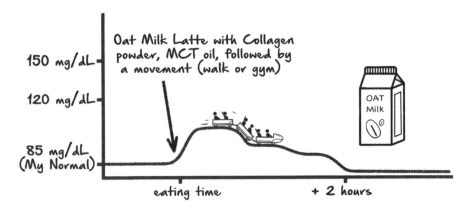

Morning smoothie inspired by a famous health guru: up 50.

Chocolate cake: up 70.

But that wasn't as surprising as eating carbs! This entire time, I thought my glucose levels were linked only to sugar, but the processed carbs (quite common in the vegan diet) impacted my glucose even more.

My favorite sourdough basil pesto zucchini toast: up 80. *#heartbroken*

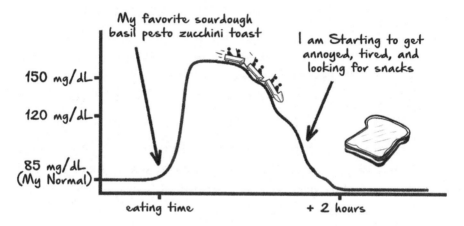

That same toast with an egg and avocado: up 54.

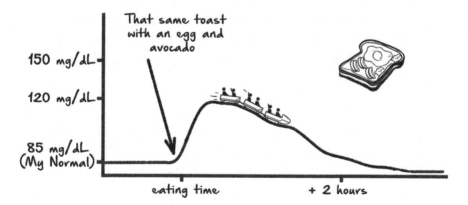

Oatmeal: up 70.

Pasta: up 80.

Pasta bolognese: up 40.

About two years into wearing the CGM, my friend Billy saw my monitor and said, "You need to meet my friend Jessie Inchauspé. She wears one, too." I looked her up and immediately felt seen and fell in love with her mission. She is now known as the Glucose Goddess and is a worldwide sensation with over 2.5 million followers and still growing as fast as a glucose spike after Skittles!

She was kind enough to share her expertise in my Fit as F*ck challenge to teach people about what glucose does to your body. At the time, however, she was just an ordinary person going through the same issues I was and sharing her findings so that people could learn from her experiences. And I'm so, so grateful that she did because it opened my eyes to huge mistakes I'd been making for years about what I thought was healthy eating.

Here's what you need to know about tackling the role of glucose in your biohacking journey. We will talk about what glucose is, how it works, why glucose spikes are harmful, and simple and practical hacks for how to manage them.

What Are Glucose Spikes and Why Should I Care?

Whenever you eat something sugary or starchy (carby), your blood sugar level can rise quickly. This is called a "glucose spike." They are completely normal and not inherently harmful; in fact, they provide immediate energy.

For a long time, the medical and scientific community thought that only diabetics should care about their glucose levels. But new studies show that the vast majority (almost 90%) of the population has unhealthy glucose spikes daily. Why? Because we as a society eat a lot of carbs and sugar, drink a lot of our calories (like juices, lattes, and sodas), and lead largely sedentary lifestyles, the glucose spikes become more frequent and more prevalent.

Unmanaged, they can give you energy crashes, age your skin, disrupt your hormones, and make you put on weight—especially around the midsection.

On top of that, When your insulin is high, your ability to burn fat cells is switched off. Even though we love our fat cells and have made peace with them, your natural ability to lose weight is locked when your insulin levels are too elevated.

For women, there's an added layer of complexity as fluctuations in blood sugar levels can also affect the menstrual cycle, potentially leading to irregular periods and fertility issues. This is why understanding and managing glucose spikes is not just about avoiding the immediate energy crash afterward but also about maintaining hormonal harmony and protecting against chronic health issues like PCOS or insulin resistance.

How Does It Feel?

How do you know when your glucose is spiking? One sure way, of course, is to use a CGM. But you don't need to wear a special device to know if you're experiencing a glucose spike—just pay attention to how your body feels. If you suddenly feel tired, thirsty, short of breath, anxious, hangry, nauseated, or if you have a dry mouth or feel like you need to go to the bathroom more often than usual, it could be a sign that your blood sugar level has spiked. A few symptoms you may experience if you are on a glucose roller coaster include:

- Feeling tired throughout the day.
- Having intense cravings for sweet foods or whatever kind of junk is around you. (The more glucose spikes you have, the more crashes occur, and then you will crave more sweets because your body is looking for fast energy. It's a vicious cycle.) That 3 p.m. slump is one sure way to tell.

- Problems with your hormones that present in symptoms like PCOS (often called diabetes of the ovaries), infertility, acne, menstrual cycle, poor sleep, and even hair loss.

During a glucose spike, the first thing that happens in your body is the mitochondria, your cell's powerhouse, become stressed out and overwhelmed, causing a release of free radicals. In other words, your cells get robbed of energy.

The second major problem with glucose spikes is that they accelerate the natural aging process, called glycation.

Glycation

In her book *Glucose Revolution*, Jessie Inchauspé explains that glycation is the process of your body browning from the inside, just like a slice of bread in the toaster. Imagine that you are born as a piece of plain white bread. When you put that piece of bread in a toaster, it gets browner and browner until it finally burns up.

That is the same with the inside of your body. When you have too much glucose in your body, it causes excess glycation, which leads to wrinkles, free radicals, and oxidative stress. Just like toast, as we get "browner" inside, we can't return to being a piece of bread. "You can't un-toast the toast," as the expression goes.

The more glucose is in your body, the more glycation occurs and, thus, more aging. Our bodies have to have a way to remove that excess glucose to avoid this. Our pancreas releases insulin that stores the glucose in the form of glycogen—first in our cells, then our liver, then our muscles. Finally, if too much glucose is still running around, it is stored in our fat cells. So by getting fatter, your body is actually saving you from toasting on the inside! (Just one more reason to send some love to those fat cells.)

Glycemic Index

To compare the impact of different foods on blood glucose levels, we can use the glycemic index to calculate the glycemic load of a food. Glycemic index (GI) is a measure of how fast a food containing carbohydrates increases your blood sugar level. Foods with a high GI are quickly absorbed by the body and can cause a rapid spike in glucose levels, while foods with a low GI are broken down more slowly, leading to a slower and more sustained rise in blood sugar levels.

High glycemic index foods include things like white bread or anything with white flour or corn, pastries, candies, crackers, starchy vegetables like potatoes, juices, energy drinks, and dried or canned fruit, as well as dates and raisins.

The Glucose Hacks

But hey, it doesn't mean you need to give up carbs and sugar whole-hog. Below, I'll share some of my favorite glucose hacks, including a few that Jessie shares in *The Glucose Revolution*. And do you know the best part? The more you use them, the fewer glucose spikes you will have, which means the less sugar and carbs you will end up craving!

It doesn't mean you won't feel like having any; it means they are going to come from a place of "I think I want a croissant today" vs. "I need a croissant because I feel like I'm dying, and I will destroy anyone standing between me and the kitchen right now."

Eat Food in the Right Order

One way to help curb glucose spikes is that, instead of restricting carbs (aka *what* you eat) like a "diet" would have you do, you will simply change the order in which you eat your food. ***Start with fiber (vegetables), then protein and fats, then carbs (starches), and finish with sugar.***

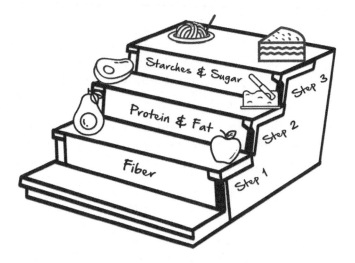

That's it. You don't need to wait 30 minutes or eat all your meals separately. You don't even have to make a sacrifice to the gods of biohacking to prevent a glucose spike.

Let me explain. Here's what a typical breakfast might look like for me: avocado, a few stalks of asparagus, a few slices of smoked salmon or some eggs, and a slice of toast. So, in this breakfast, I would:

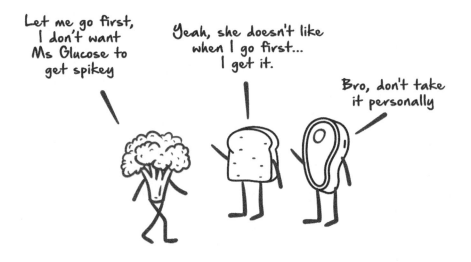

Eat my fiber first: Start with vegetables, such as avocado, asparagus, or other leafy greens.

Secondly, proteins: Next would follow my eggs, bacon, or salmon.

Finish with starches: This is where I would have my toast, if I am having some. This is also the place to have some whole fruit. Make sure any carbohydrates—starches and sugars (even if they contain a lot of fiber, like apples)—are eaten last!

Now, that doesn't mean you can't mix your food. I usually start with veggies as the first few bites, almost like an appetizer. I then add my eggs and salmon to the mix. After I finish most of my plate, I start nibbling on the toast.

Eat Those Veggies First

I remember when I didn't want to finish dinner growing up. My mom always said, "Have some vegetables and meat first, then you can eat the rest." Mom knew I only wanted to eat the rest (potatoes). But it turns out that Mom was right (as usual). Eating fiber (aka vegetables) first can have huge health benefits.

Vegetables are full of fiber that your body can't absorb or break down.

Think of fiber as a sponge. When you eat your veggies first, they slow down the absorption of glucose in your digestive tract by soaking much of it up. Fiber is also like a scrub brush, cleaning out bacteria and other buildup so you will have a healthier gut and possibly reduce your risk of small intestinal bacterial overgrowth (SIBO) or cancer.

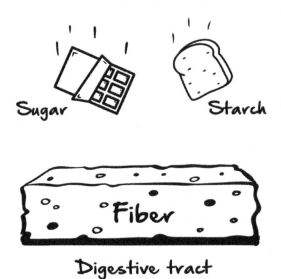

Digestive tract

I like to munch on carrots and celery while I cook, getting some fiber into my system before I even sit down to eat. Some other ideas for fiber starters might include:

- Sliced raw vegetables: cucumbers, zucchini (and, of course, carrots and celery)
- Olives
- Grilled or roasted artichoke with lemon and olive oil dip
- Cruciferous vegetables like cauliflower, broccoli, and brussels sprouts
- Kimchi or pickles

Fats and Proteins Second

After eating some vegetables, eat your fats and proteins next. Protein is found in meat, fish, eggs, and dairy products, while fat is found in coconut or olive oil, butter, and avocados. Because of their low glycemic index (meaning they are low in sugars), proteins and fats can be digested without being impacted by a spike in insulin because they do not trigger a high insulin response. Like fiber, they also slow absorption, making you feel fuller for longer and lowering glucose levels.

Finish with Your Carbs & Sugar

Finally, always have your carbs (in other words, starches and sugars) last. You are much more likely to already be near-full and satisfied by the time you get to them, which means you can feel content without giving in to consuming a large amount of carbs. Eating these last reduces glucose levels by 75 percent, which slows down the aging and weight-gain process significantly!

This one little veggies-protein-carbs (VPC) trick can be a total game changer for your blood sugar levels, keeping those cravings at bay and keeping you feeling satisfied for longer. Plus, your digestive system will be doing a happy dance.

And the best part? Did you notice that nothing was cut out of your diet and no calories were counted? You can kiss goodbye to the days of ditching your favorite treats or wallowing in the nagging guilt that follows. It's all about smart, stress-free biohacking.

Here's a biohack. You may have heard that cooling down cooked rice (or other starchy foods) and then reheating the dish later turns it from a "simple carb" to a "complex carb." This isn't exactly correct, but cooling down your rice, pasta, or potatoes increases their resistant starch content, so it won't be digested and absorbed as quickly. Remember, this is a good thing in biohacking. Resistant starch acts similarly to dietary fiber in the body. It "resists" digestion in the small intestine and proceeds to the large intestine, where it can act as food for beneficial gut bacteria. So, while the basic starch structure in rice doesn't change, cooling and then reheating will help your blood sugar.

Have Green Calories Before All Your Meals

Counting calories is so old school, and research shows that one calorie is not equal to another. Calories in a food tell you nothing about what the food is made of and what it's doing to your body—like whether or not it's creating a glucose spike. A hundred calories of broccoli and a hundred calories of chocolate are completely different. You can eat more calories than somebody else and lose more weight than them if you're eating in a way that doesn't spike your glucose levels. Adding extra greens before each meal will help you feel fuller for longer, reduce your cravings, and lower your glucose levels.

For example, say you and your bestie have pasta, but you ate a 200-calorie salad beforehand. Technically, you consumed more calories than her, but you'll likely achieve your fitness goals faster because the extra fiber before your dinner will change the way your body digests and processes the pasta.

As I write this, I'm just about to leave the house to meet my friend for lunch. I know we're going to have pizza, so I am about to employ a little hack that I've been living by that has been super helpful for me to enjoy my life and indulge in carbs.

Obviously, eating carbs, especially ones like pizza, would give me a huge spike. Before I leave the house (or at the restaurant if that is an option), I will have some salad to give me a fiber base. I usually add some carrot sticks or olives to up the fiber quotient. You could also add some apple cider vinegar dressing with olive oil to the salad or drink it with some water to help it go down a bit easier. With just a little bit of fiber first, you can have any starches you want without getting a horrendous glucose spike. The only thing to remember is that you have a two-hour window after eating the fiber to enjoy those carbs or sugars.

Apple Cider Vinegar—the Magic Elixir

So what happens when you don't fancy vegetables and feel like having that chocolate fudge at 4 p.m.? Well, you can have a tablespoon of apple cider vinegar (ACV) diluted in a glass of water. It is such an excellent glucose hack that I use it every day. Add a tablespoon or two of apple cider vinegar (be sure it is organic and filtered), stir it in a large glass of water, throw it back, and then indulge.

Apple cider vinegar lowers your glucose spikes by up to 30%. It can help with weight loss by promoting feelings of fullness, reducing appetite, and aiding in the breakdown of fats.

On top of that, ACV contains acetic acid, which aids digestion. It seems counterintuitive, but if you suffer from acid reflux, indigestion, heartburn, or any of those not-so-sexy digestive issues, a lot of times, your body is too alkaline. Try ACV before your meal and see how you feel. The more acidic your digestive tract is, the more effectively minerals, nutrients, and (especially important for women) calcium are absorbed.

ACV also helps you hold on to potassium, a powerful mineral in our bodies. Plus, ACV has antimicrobial properties and can stop the growth of harmful bacteria, such as E. coli.

ACV is like Beyoncé, Taylor Swift, Selena Gomez, and Eleanor Roosevelt all rolled up into one. It can do almost anything a modern woman could want for her body (it also helps acne and gives hair shine!), but it isn't some new discovery; it's been under our noses and in our pantries for years.

Does this mean that you should have apple cider vinegar with every meal, since it sounds like a magical cure-all? Would you want Eleanor Roosevelt sitting across from you at every single meal? I mean, she's amazing, but at some point, you might want to talk about something other than the fight for human rights in the 1930s and

1940s. Is this an important topic? Absolutely. But it's probably the most impactful in strategic doses.

Remember: too much of a good thing is not a good thing. ACV is highly acidic, consuming it undiluted or in large amounts can erode tooth enamel over time. (You can prevent this by always diluting ACV in a glass of water, drinking it through a straw, rinsing your mouth with water afterward, or taking it in pill form, like we have available at Biohacking Bestie). Drinking too much ACV may also lead to irritation or damage to the esophagus or cause other issues like stomach upset, bloating, or diarrhea, especially when taken in large quantities.

I know that some of my students can't bring themselves to drink ACV as it makes them gag. I noticed that unless ACV is organic and with the "mother" (the mix of yeast and good bacteria resulting from the fermentation process), I also find it hard to drink. But remember: If you can't choke it down, don't. I believe in your body's intelligence, and if she says, "I don't want it," don't force her. She knows best.

Right Order During the Day

Breakfast has some of the most culturally conditioned foods out there. When I am at my house in Bali, locals have rice for breakfast. In Poland, my parents start the day with a ham and cheese sandwich; in Los Angeles, it seems like everyone has a smoothie! I am writing this chapter while sitting in a cafe in Paris, and the server just asked me, "Would you like to have a French croissant or American egg-and-sausage breakfast?"

I know how much it takes to create a new breakfast routine. It's hard to change how we eat, but breakfast is extra hard for some reason. Maybe you hate eggs or love smoothies, in which case, you're not going to like what I am about to tell you, which is one of my few hard and fast rules: Your breakfast needs to be savory (aka not sweet).

I know I promised you that you wouldn't have to say farewell to your favorite foods, and I wasn't lying. When it comes to oatmeal, pastries, pancakes, and donuts, you can still have them—just not as breakfast. As a dessert later in the day? Go for it. But it won't serve you well first thing in the morning.

Always Start Your Day with a Savory Breakfast

Meet two sisters; let's call them Annabelle and Kate. Both sisters eat the same food throughout the day: yogurt with granola, avocado toast, eggs, steak, veggies, and some bread. Everything is alike except that they eat it differently.

Kate starts her day with an oat milk latte, followed by yogurt with granola and fruit for breakfast. She has an avocado toast with eggs and a salad for lunch, then wraps it up with a steak and veggies for dinner. Kate eats a very healthy version of a standard American diet: sweet breakfast, light lunch, and protein-heavy dinner.

Annabelle, on the other hand, starts her day with eggs, avocados, and a salad (after fasting according to her cycle, which you will learn too!) She then has an oat milk latte. For lunch, she has steak and veggies followed by yogurt with granola and fruit as a dessert. For dinner, Annabelle goes out with her friends and has some pasta with chicken. Technically, Annabelle had one extra meal.

Which one of them will have more energy and lose weight faster? Well, here is the wild part: Even though Annabelle had more calories, she will lose weight faster, have more energy throughout the day, and feel better all around than Kate.

Why? Well, mostly because she ate her food in the right order throughout the day, especially starting her morning with a high-protein breakfast.

Breakfast time is when we quite literally *"break our fasts."* Whenever you break a fast, your blood sugars (i.e., glucose levels) will naturally rise. You want to ensure they rise in a steady, controlled manner rather than causing a huge spike (and subsequent crash) in your glucose levels.

After you haven't eaten for a long time (like overnight), your body is waiting in the starting blocks for you to start eating. It's naturally more insulin sensitive. Do you know how you like to start your morning gently with some soft mantras in the background instead of heavy rock or scream therapy? It's like that, except it's your guts and sugar.

If you start your day with simple, processed carbs (like oat milk), the glucose will skyrocket, like the Burj Khalifa in Dubai. We already mentioned earlier you always want to start eating your meals with fiber, but it's even truer for breakfast. Fiber is like a sponge or a mesh net that catches the glucose and prevents it from hitting your gut.

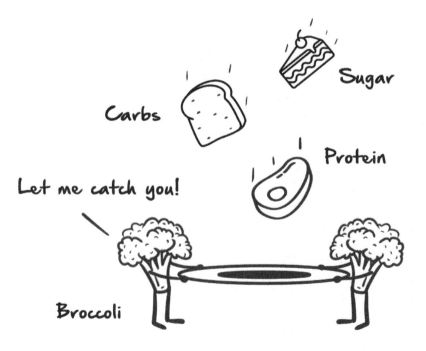

This is why having protein and fat, plus lots of fiber, for breakfast is a fantastic strategy for breaking your fast. It aids in blood sugar control, supports gut health, facilitates a quicker shift to a fat-burning state, and helps maintain hormonal balance. It's a win on multiple levels! Just remember to keep variety in your vegetable fiber sources to feed different types of beneficial bacteria in your gut.

When you have a sweet breakfast, you are signing yourself up for huge spikes in glucose that will make it very hard for your body to enter fat-burning mode because they will trigger more insulin production.

A savory breakfast (think eggs, proteins, nuts, avocados, or other good fats) that is low in sugar will allow you to avoid that spike in glucose! If you have a big glucose spike at breakfast, your whole day will kick off that glucose roller coaster, and you will crave sugar every couple of hours to maintain that high and stave off the inevitable crash just a little bit longer. Keeping glucose levels steady prevents the crazy cravings, plus your energy improves, your hormones start to regulate, and you set yourself up for better long-term health by preventing conditions like diabetes.

Look, I know that a latte or fancy iced coffee is the one thing you don't hate about your morning commute. I feel you, and I promise I wouldn't be asking this of you if I didn't know that a drink like that on an empty stomach is setting you up for a massive glucose spike and crash. If you *really* only want the coffee, try switching from regular sugar to monk fruit as a sweetener, which doesn't raise your blood glucose.

I tell you what: how about we compromise? You agree to try some of the hacks we've discussed, and I agree not to say, "I told you so," when you have so much more energy throughout the rest of your day.

P.S.—Not ready to divorce your oat milk latte first thing in the morning? Add unflavored collagen peptides (protein) and a drop of MCT oil (good fat) to reduce the glucose spike.

Breakfast Food That Should Never Be Breakfast Food

America has it backward. We are bombarded with sweet breakfast options that set us up for more snacking later on during the day. Here are some breakfast foods that shouldn't be, despite their marketing.

Sugary cereals and granola: Many breakfast cereals are high in added sugars and low in fiber and protein.

Pastries: Donuts, croissants, and muffins are often high in sugar, processed flour, and unhealthy fats like trans fats, which are particularly harmful to heart health.

Prepackaged breakfast sandwiches or burritos: These can be high in sodium and unhealthy fats and often contain processed meats.

All the sugar and flour combos: Biscuits, breakfast sandwiches, pancakes, French toast, crepes, waffles—you name it. Please avoid these, especially when they are covered with processed sugar like high fructose corn syrup.

Sugary drinks: Drinks like prepackaged drinks and flavored coffees can be loaded with added sugars. Sorry, Starbucks salted caramel latte. You are delicious and I honor you for that, but you don't deserve to be the first thing I put into my mouth in the morning.

Flavored, fat-free yogurts: These are either full of sugar or artificial sweeteners and emulsifiers to compensate for the absolute lack of taste that fat-free foods have.

Smoothies and fruit juices: While I agree the nutritional value of smoothies is pretty good, any kind of fruit combo, when blended with milk and possibly sweetened sugar or honey, will give you a massive glucose spike. I'm all for smoothies, just as a dessert.

Instead of these breakfast imposters, a better alternative would be to build a savory breakfast around protein, and kick it off with some vegetables to supply your fiber. Think along these lines:

- A sliced avocado topped with crispy, crumbled, pasture-raised bacon and a sprinkle of sea salt
- Soft-boiled eggs with wild-caught salmon
- Egg white omelet with mushrooms
- Homemade baked egg muffins
- Zucchini "noodles" with pesto and soft-boiled eggs
- Savory smoothie bowl like my favorite avocado chocolate

Have a Dessert as a Dessert

Another glucose rule is that dessert should stay as a true dessert, not become a bedtime snack. Back in the day, I would have dinner or lunch and wait a couple of hours to have my favorite key lime pie or apple pie as a separate meal. It was *terrible* for my glucose. It turns out it's better to have that sweet treat right at the end of a meal rather than waiting two or three hours before having something sugary. If you eat your treat by itself, guess what will happen? That's right. You can say it with me by now: It will cause a glucose spike, and glucose spikes lead to … (wait for it) … *even more cravings*!

I should add that this end-of-meal time is also the best time to have fruit if you desire it. Even though fruit has some beneficial nutrients, it still has fructose and will increase your glucose. Whole fruit does have fiber in it, so the fiber will help your body process the glucose more slowly than drinking fruit juice, but you still want to treat it as a dessert and enjoy it at the end of your meal.

Interestingly, if you consume fructose, your body can't store it anywhere except in your fat cells, debunking the myth that dietary fat makes you fat. It isn't eating fat that makes you fat, it's the fructose and your body's inability to store it anywhere other than fat cells. Fructose is found in many processed items such as fruit juices, sauces, sodas, high fructose corn syrup, salad dressings, and dried fruit.

When we are working out, our body uses up the storage from the liver and the muscles first, and when that is used up, it starts pulling from the fat cells. But this process can't happen if your insulin levels are too high because the cells become locked and can't release the fat. To lose weight, you need to keep your glucose levels low and steady so those fat cells can open and you can burn fat. Otherwise, you can work out as much as you want, and you still won't lose weight. I know that is not what you wanted to hear, but don't blame the messenger. I'm on *your* side, remember?

Sugar Needs Wing Men

Now, sugar is a troublemaker who doesn't know how to behave in your gut, so never send it unsupervised. What do I mean? If I have my favorite apple pie alone, my glucose will spike like crazy. The same goes for toast. But if I have my toast with avocado (healthy fat) or butter (which is basic but delicious), my spike isn't as bad because the sugar isn't running around my gut all alone. That means adding some nuts to your oatmeal, Greek yogurt to your cake, or butter to your pastry can actually help your body process the sugar more effectively. (Did I just encourage you to put *more butter* on your pastry? Why, yes. Yes, I did. You're welcome.)

KEY TAKEAWAYS

- Constant fluctuations in blood sugar can impact your hormones, potentially leading to issues like PCOS and insulin resistance.

- Recognizing glucose spikes can be done by paying attention to symptoms like tiredness, cravings for sweets, and hormonal imbalances.

- Glucose spikes stress cells and accelerate the aging process through glycation.

- The glycemic index (GI) measures how quickly foods with carbohydrates raise blood sugar levels.

- Fructose can only be stored in fat cells, so managing glucose levels is crucial for weight loss.

- Eat Food in the Right Order: Start with fiber (vegetables), then protein and fats, and finish with carbs and sugar.

- Have Green Calories Before All Your Meals: Adding greens before meals can reduce cravings and lower glucose levels.

- Apple Cider Vinegar (ACV): ACV can lower glucose spikes by up to 30% and aid digestion but should be consumed in moderation.

- Right Order During the Day: Start the day with a savory, high-protein breakfast to control glucose levels and maintain hormonal balance.

- Dessert as a Dessert: Enjoy sweets as part of a meal, not as a stand-alone snack.

- Sugar Needs Wing Men: Combining sugar with healthy fats or protein can help the body process it more effectively.

CHAPTER 3

HOW TO FAST LIKE THE QUEEN YOU ARE

Fasting Tips and Tricks

I probably shouldn't say this, but you can stay on the not-so-great SAD (Standard American Diet) and still see massive improvements to your health just with fasting alone! *(Gasp! I know, right?)*

Also, eating the same number of calories within a shorter time frame can lead to weight loss, plain and simple. Fasting increases your metabolic rate by 3.6-14%, helping you burn more calories throughout the day without sending your body into panic mode. It's like giving your body's calorie-burning engine a little tune-up.

When I was vegan, I had my first breakfast at 6 a.m. when I woke up (toast with almond butter and a banana), another piece of toast and a smoothie at 8 a.m. after my workout, then oatmeal at 11 a.m. That's right—I had three breakfasts before noon. That's more breakfasts than a hobbit. Great as it sounds, though, the triple breakfast method keeps you obsessed with food, weak, and grumpy! Let's try something better, shall we?

Micro-fasting: Don't Snack!

Let's start small. Fasting literally means to "go without." You can go without food, social media, negative thoughts, and even your toxic ex. In a society where all we do is constantly consume (social media, another latte, Netflix), the idea of fasting from something is a beautiful spiritual practice.

Now, just like a pair of jeans, fasting does not fit everyone (unless you're in a magical YA novel about traveling pants). It may not be for you if you have a history of disordered eating, are pregnant, or are going through a particularly stressful time in life. Biohacking is about prioritizing your health, so that's what you need to do right now.

But, as your biohacking bestie, I would love for you to give "micro-fasts" a try. These are suitable for everyone. Micro-fasts are simply when you give your body at least three hours of rest between putting things into your mouth (besides plain tea and water).

Aggie, I barely have time to pee between my morning meetings, let alone make a meal. I know! See how easy this is? Chances are, you already have a micro-fast or two built into your day. Good job! Keep going!

There are many fitness meal plans that suggest eating up to seven snacks a day—just grabbing a little handful of something healthy whenever you have a free moment so that your body never reaches the point where it is hungry. But a little hunger is good. Later in the chapter, I'll introduce you to leptin and ghrelin, the two hormones that make you feel "hungry" and "full." For now, though, I would love for you to unlearn snacking if that's a habit for you.

Want to know something interesting? Snacking throughout the day is an invention of the 1980s processed food companies who were trying to increase their markets by changing human behavior by convincing you that you needed to have bars, chips, smoothies, and lattes close at hand to make it through life.

And we never stop consuming. From a morning coffee to that Insta-gram reel, you are bombarding your body with information, food, and drinks. Unfortunately, when it comes to consuming snacks, not only is this constant consumption leading you to take in more calories, it also doesn't give your gut a rest. Your body needs about two hours to digest a meal fully, and if you start consuming calories again during that time (yes, liquids too), you disrupt this process.

Imagine a caboose (your Migrating Motor Complex, or MMC) trans-porting the food from your stomach to the lower intestine; this takes about 90-120 minutes. Every time you eat again during that time frame, the caboose has to come back up your intestine, which can overwhelm your body and may be the reason why you get bloated.

Practicing at least two micro-fasts, three hours long, each day can drastically change your eating patterns and how your body responds to them.

The F-A-S-T Framework

My friend Jessica was determined to try fasting but was frustrated at her lack of progress. Like everyone else in LA, she enjoyed her oat milk latte in the morning, "And then I have nothing until 2 p.m.," she said. "But I just see no results. Fasting is useless."

I didn't know how to "break it" to Jessica that she had already bro-ken her fast (see what I did there?) when she downed that latte, and, at that point, she would have been better off eating a big ol' savory breakfast. You know the saying, "Breakfast like a king, lunch like a prince, dinner like a pauper." Make your breakfast count.

Fast forward to four months later, and Jessica has lost 10 kg (over 20 lbs) and recently messaged me: "I never knew I could lose the stub-born fat; I always thought I would be a bigger girl. I trained with the best personal trainers. None of them gave me the results that fasting the right way did. I always craved a big breakfast with eggs and bacon but judged myself for it because I saw other girls having smoothies and looking great. But I always felt bloated after smoothies. I feel like a new person thanks to fasting."

As biohack(h)ers, we love fasting because it regulates hormones, improves insulin sensitivity, increases the growth hormone (the one that keeps you looking young like Jennifer Lopez), removes toxins through autophagy, and reduces inflammation.

Here is my FAST acronym for Biohacking Queens:

F: Feast

It may be counterintuitive, but fasting without feasting is starvation, which is especially true for women because we often forget that too much of a good thing is not always better! Most women follow fasting protocols created for men and can end up skipping their periods, noticing their hair getting weak, and then (understandably) calling the whole fasting thing a scam. It's not, but you have to know how to fast like a woman, and for women, less is often more when it comes to fasting. We will learn how to fast according to your cycle in Chapter 6.

A: Adjust and Adapt

Fasting is a stressor for your body. It's a good one, but it is still a stressor. If you don't get enough sleep or have a lot of demands at work, pushing yourself at a gym on an empty stomach will not make you feel safe, resulting in your stress hormone (cortisol) spiking, which in turn causes you to gain weight and feel on-edge and overwhelmed. We want to make sure you adjust and adapt your fasting every single day to your circumstances, and sometimes the best way to fast is ... not at all.

S: Slow

When I climbed Kilimanjaro, the highest peak in Africa, my guide would repeat *"polepole"* all the time, which means "slower" in

Swahili. Often, I see my students learn about the benefits of fasting and then the next day—having never fasted before—attempt to do it for 17 to 20 hours. *Please don't.* Seriously, don't. If you are new to fasting, try delaying your breakfast by 20 minutes in the morning. That's it. Do this every other day, and stop seven days before your period (or as close as you can approximate if your cycles aren't super regular). Then have an earlier dinner. Again, not five hours earlier, just 20 minutes earlier. You will be able to fast for much longer in no time and without unnecessary pain. Going to extreme measures (and feeling miserable while you do it) right off the bat will make you disillusioned with this whole process reeeeaaaally quickly. *Polepole*, mama.

T: Timing

Timing is key. As a woman, you can't go without food whenever. You want to fast according to your cycle so you don't disrupt your hormones. Also, an earlier dinner is better than having a super late breakfast. A good rule of thumb for me is that I don't eat after sunset or less than three hours before going to sleep. Digestion will disrupt the quality of your sleep, and sleep is your anti-aging super tool.

Wanna Carrot?

How do you know if you are hungry? It may sound like a silly question, but most of us take a craving or dehydration for hunger and run to the fridge as if we are about to die. I promise you're not. Next time you feel ready to eat, try the carrot test! If someone handed you a beautiful carrot to eat, would you eat it? If the answer is yes, you are hungry. If you don't think the carrot looks appealing and all you want is a scoop of ice cream instead, this is a craving.

With cravings, you feel like you have no control. They are usually head-driven, motivated by thoughts, feelings, or emotions. You go by the grocery store bakery, and you have to have something sweet. It usually is a desire for a specific food or flavor like sweet or salty, chocolate, or chips. Many women equate sugary or starchy foods as comfort foods if they are anxious, stressed, or bored. Cravings can also be a sign of candida in your gut, a glucose crash, or an inadequate diet.

When you are *actually* hungry, your body releases a hormone called ghrelin that gives you a feeling of hunger. It's the "feed me" hormone, when your stomach growls and you may feel lightheaded or hangry. When your body releases ghrelin, it starts a chain reaction that allows you to go into the fat cells to release some of the fat stored in them for energy. If you don't allow yourself to feel hungry, you won't allow your body to use up the fat storage (I'll explain it in detail in a moment).

Many biohackers or experts would tell you to exercise for 20 minutes after the first signs of hunger to boost your fat burning, and I absolutely agree. Some amount of hunger is good for your body as long as you don't go to the point of starving.

So here is the biohack: When you start to feel *hungry*, if you are able to go on a quick 20-minute walk, you can maximize your body's fat-burning capacity. Next time you feel a *craving*, have some water and some good fat! I've noticed that when I crave sugar, what I really need is more good fat like butter, olive oil, or even cocoa. Try offering your body some avocado and see if she doesn't calm down and allow you to release that craving.

Fasting Shouldn't Feel Like Dying

I was standing in the kitchen washing the dishes and listening to a Dave Asprey podcast when I heard, "Fasting shouldn't feel like you're dying."

"Bullshit," I said out loud, like the delicate flower I am. My brain immediately started ranting at him: *I just attempted a 24-hour fast, and five hours in my stomach was in soooo much pain, I had brain fog, and I stayed a whole day in bed in a state of deep misery. I can't believe people fast like this every day. What a terrible, miserable life.*

Dave continued, "If you can't go for more than three to four hours without food, it means you don't have metabolic flexibility, and it's beautiful feedback for you to know your diet sucks for you."

Wait—this sounds rational. Dammit. Okay, sorry, Dave, I take that back. Also, I don't have what? Metabolic flexibility? What is that? Am I trying to keep my metabolism from pulling a hammy? This sounds bananas, but also ... tell me more.

It turns out your metabolic flexibility is, in fact, a real thing, and it has everything to do with how your body burns energy.

Two Metabolisms Are Better than One

Did you know you have not one, but two metabolisms? And did you know that you can switch between the two as a pretty sure way of helping you lose weight? Whaaaaaa? *I know.* We're gonna get a little sciency for a moment, but hear me out because there are a few terms I need you to become besties with as a biohack(h)er.

Picture this: We're hanging out in the backyard of the house that is your body. When I say we "burn" calories, I mean it: it's like you have a furnace or firepit going back there. What do you put into the bonfire? Logs, twigs, and maybe some paper to start it with.

When I say you have two different metabolisms, you can run on a mix of two fuels: carbohydrates (carbs) and fats. Carbs are like quick-burning twigs, while fats are like slow-burning logs. When you eat a lot of carbs, your body uses them as the primary fuel source. It's like throwing a bunch of twigs into the fire. They burn quickly, giving you a burst of energy, but it also doesn't last long. You need to keep adding more twigs to keep the fire going. This is how most people live: using twigs for energy. Twigs are handy and your body loves them.

Ketosis

When you fast for longer than 17 hours, however, your body runs out of twigs. This is also true when you reduce your carb intake significantly, like going on a low-carb or ketogenic diet.

At this point, she starts looking for an alternative fuel source. She's like: *there are these beautiful big logs stored away that I could use for energy, but they are stored all the way in the fat cells, which is a pain.* So she takes her sweet time before she gets them (about 16 hours since your last meal). However, the moment your body starts using logs (ketones) instead of twigs, you are in ketosis.

Fat Adaptation

Ketosis is not the same as fat adaptation. Ketosis is the initial process where your body starts producing and using ketones for fuel. It's like learning to burn logs instead of twigs to sustain the fire. On the other hand, fat adaptation is like becoming a master at burning logs. Over time, as your body becomes more efficient at using fats as fuel, it becomes fat-adapted, meaning that it knows the ropes so well it doesn't need the big lead-up time to get into that mode. It's like having a well-stocked woodpile that keeps the fire going for a long time without needing constant refueling.

Metabolic Flexibility

Metabolic flexibility is your ability to switch from burning twigs (carbs) to burning logs (fat). What science is now realizing is that the more you switch between the two metabolisms, the easier it's going to be for you to burn the fat that has been "impossible" to lose, to feel more energetic, and to make your body more insulin sensitive (all the things we want).

Autophagy, the Marie Kondo of Your Body

Meet Autophagy (pronounced as "aw-TOFF-uh-jee"), the Marie Kondo of your body. After 17 hours of fasting, when your body wants to get the logs, autophagy goes to the basement (and if you are new to fasting, this is the first time she has done much of anything in a long time). There will be so much clutter along the way because no one has been down there for years!

Imagine your cells are like rooms in a house. Over time, things start to pile up—worn-out proteins, dysfunctional parts, and a heap of other "junky" heavy metals. This is where autophagy steps in, and like the reality-TV-star-turned-cleaning-guru Marie Kondo, she asks the simple question, "Does it spark joy?"

She cleans the house, tidying everything up and throwing away the trash, thinking, "This trash is leaking my energy; I don't want to keep it here." Sometimes she decides to give certain cells another life, like a good pair of old jeans, and finds a way to reuse and recycle them.

Just look at this amazing resource you've carried with you all these years, but if you've never fasted, you've never gotten to meet her. Autophagy is linked with longevity and is a natural defense against diseases like cancer, infections, and inflammatory diseases because of the intense cleaning, clearing, and reorganizing she does. She also improves muscle performance, enhances weight loss, and boosts mood. All that to say, autophagy should be your new best friend *(besides me)*.

What Breaks a Fast

So, if fasting is so important, let's take a second to think about what breaks a fast. The simple answer is any type of solid food; drinks that contain calories, such as any type of milk (yes, even oat, coconut, and almond); coconut water; juices; alcohol; and most kinds of coffee drinks or tea with added milk, sugar, honey, or cream. Although they claim to be calorie-free, diet drinks filled with artificial sweeteners will only hurt your fast because they trick your body into thinking you are consuming sugar. Your body will respond to the artificial sugar as if it is regular sugar and release the same chemicals in response. That means those water flavor additives that are "zero calories" should not be put in your water while fasting.

What Doesn't Break a Fast?

Pure water does not contain calories and is crucial for staying hydrated, especially during a longer fast.

Black coffee (as long as no milk, sugar, or cream is added) is okay unless you fast for gut purposes. One exception is bulletproof coffee (black coffee with butter and MCT oil). Even though it technically breaks your fast because it has calories, it will kick you into ketosis and make you less hungry. It's an excellent biohack to get all the benefits of fasting without being hungry!

Apple cider vinegar with a drop of lemon when you wake up is a fantastic way to start your day, whether fasting or not.

Most supplements, like vitamins, minerals, (and Biohacking Bestie products), do not contain calories and therefore do not typically break a fast.

Buffer Hack

I know that for my mom, who is 65, making drastic diet changes doesn't sound very exciting. She doesn't want to start her day any differently than she does now. A cup of coffee with oat milk and a sandwich. She doesn't want to give up, either.

But she doesn't have to! Remember—this is not 1s and 0s.

If this sounds like you, please remember you don't have to give up anything, either. My suggestions are merely a few "buffer" biohacks. Try these for a few weeks and see how you feel:

1. Before your coffee, have a glass of water with 1-2 tablespoons of ACV and a little squeeze of lemon.

2. Have your coffee ten minutes later than usual. Not more. Then, add some unflavored grass-fed collagen peptides (which we offer at Biohacking Bestie) and a drop of MCT oil to your coffee. I promise you will barely even know they're there; they won't change the taste and will make your coffee a little creamier, but the protein and healthy fat will be a much better way of starting your morning, especially if you drink oat milk.

3. Add some "green calories" (such as extra vegetables) to your sandwich. Maybe it's avocado; maybe it's cucumber or homegrown sprouts. Actually adding more good green calories will help your hormones.

That's it. You aren't making any drastic changes—you are just adding a few "buffer" biohacks that will help minimize the impact of the current non-negotiables.

P.S. My mom has lost 30 lbs in the last six months and counting from these "buffer" hacks, so there is that, too!

KEY TAKEAWAYS

- Fasting can improve health significantly, even without dietary changes, by increasing metabolic rate and promoting weight loss through calorie restriction within a shorter time frame, however it is not fit for every woman.

- Micro-fasting, which involves going without eating for a few hours, is a great practice for most people, aiding digestion and reducing calorie intake.

- The "F-A-S-T" framework for fasting helps you remember the importance of Feasting (eating well during nonfasting periods), Adjusting fasting to daily circumstances, Starting slowly, and considering Timing in relation to one's menstrual cycle for women.

- Understanding hunger versus cravings is crucial in fasting; genuine hunger signals the need for food, while cravings are often emotion-driven and can be mitigated by healthier choices like water or good fats.

- Fasting shouldn't be painful or exhausting; it's about metabolic flexibility and finding a balance that works for individual lifestyles and health conditions, including using biohacks like buffers for gradual adaptation.

- Autophagy, similar to Marie Kondo's cleaning method, is a process that begins after about 17 hours of fasting. It acts like a deep cleaning for your body's cells, removing old proteins, dysfunctional components, and heavy metals. This process is beneficial for longevity, disease prevention, improving muscle performance, enhancing weight loss, and boosting mood.

- Consuming solid food, calorie-containing drinks (including milk alternatives, juices, and alcohol), and drinks with sugar or artificial sweeteners can break a fast. Pure water, black coffee (without additives), and apple cider vinegar with lemon don't break a fast. Certain supplements also don't interfere with fasting.

- Buffer biohacks for easing into fasting: try simple biohacks like drinking water with apple cider vinegar and lemon before coffee, delaying coffee intake, and adding collagen peptides and MCT oil to coffee. These small changes can minimize the impact of dietary non-negotiables and help in gradual weight loss.

LEVEL 2:
WHAT TO EAT

CHAPTER 4

EATING IN THE REAL WORLD

Y ou've got the "when" (and it's really not that bad, is it? I hate to say, "I told you so," but ... just kidding. You're doing great. Let's keep going!) Now, let's move to the next level and look at the "what."

Only after you feel fluent in Level 1 is it time for Level 2. It's a little bit like learning Italian in school and feeling all good with a few phrases you can use in your classroom, and then you go to Rome and a waiter asks what you'd like to order and you freak out!

We are getting more advanced here, and we'll be talking about macros, toxins, and beyond, so if any of this overwhelms you at any point, please feel free to go back to Level 1 and hang out there a bit longer until you feel more confident. In fact, there is no shame in staying there forever. Truly.

I want the Biohacking Eating Lifestyle™ to be easy to follow and easy to commit to because the changes most diets bring are usually too drastic and don't fit naturally into your environment, your culture, and/or your family life! Let's be honest, when one person in a family is on a diet, suddenly everyone else is too, in one way or another, whether they want to be or not. And if everyone around you is in open rebellion about whatever new diet trend you are trying, it's going to be harder to integrate it seamlessly into your life in a way that reduces the amount of thought you give to food rather than adding to it.

I watched my mom go to different dietitians throughout my childhood, sticking to the strict meal plan for a few weeks, eating separately from me and my sister, only to come back to her favorite foods that were native to our culture and our family.

My mom's plan wasn't to become the next Cindy Crawford (to me she already was anyway!); she just wanted to feel a little better and lighter in her body, but starting a new diet every few weeks that involved restrictions, preparation stress, and family ostracism only spiked her cortisol, the stress hormone, which prevented her from losing the weight she was trying to shed by implementing all those changes.

Intro to Level 2

I want you to imagine your favorite homemade dish of all time—one you grew up loving and dreaming about. Come on, close your eyes and try to recall the smell, the texture, the taste, the temperature when it hits your tongue. Is it warm and fluffy? Or so spicy that it makes your eyes water? My favorite dish was cold pasta with strawberries, sour cream, and sugar. In fact, to this day, I eat strawberries and coconut cream daily. I don't want to live a life without strawberries and cream. No thanks. Uh-uh. Hard pass. This is one of my great joys in life.

Yet every diet plan I ever tried, not surprisingly, did not include my favorite dish in the world. I would go on a strict regimen only to give up the whole thing out of absolute misery sooner than later. Because what is life without your favorite foods?

Now, let's go back to yours. What is that favorite dish? Tiramisu? Apple pie? Pasta? What if I told you you can eat your favorite dishes—your comfort foods and core staples—almost every day and still lose weight ... provided you follow my preferences below? It's not wishful thinking; I have the science to prove it.

Biohacking Eating Lifestyle™

The Biohacking Eating Lifestyle is based on a simple principle: you deserve the best in life, full stop. As women, we are programmed by society to settle, to give way, to compromise. Not anymore.

If you are anything like me, you absolutely hate being told what to do. So the only hard and fast thing I am going to tell you to do is this: listen to yourself.

Just listen to yourself.

Take time to reconnect with your Higher Self, remember who the f*ck you are, and act (and eat) accordingly. Doesn't that sound great? The lifestyle is easy to maintain when on the go or traveling (this is coming from someone who is away from home more than 300 days a year!). It's a new lens for how to view food, not just a fad diet that will get forgotten next month. You and I have completely different histories of where we have lived and traveled, what water we drank, who we kissed, and what animals or pets we were in contact with. Add this plus our unique DNA (which predicts how well we metabolize saturated fat, coffee, or absorb certain vitamins), and all these things have an impact on how our gut, with its unique biosphere, is doing (coincidentally, we only share 10% of our gut DNA with others) and what diet would make us thrive. So, while I am sharing with you what science says, please remember you know what's best for you.

Why Do I Call These Preferences, Not Principles?

You and I don't need any more rules.

Rules are stressful, rigid, don't fit everyone, and if you miss one, you'll feel like something is wrong with you. There is not! You're living in the 2020s, and eating real food is dang hard, okay? I want to take the concept of "doing something wrong" off the table. Remember, I want you to be both a biohacker *and* bio-*slacker.* In fact, in my own life, when I eat something that's not in line with my preferences, I say to myself, "Aggie the bio-slacker is out. Good luck, liver," and laugh it off.

Also, remember that "preferences" suggest I am always free to choose. Don't cage yourself with another rule someone presented to you, even if it's me.

For example, if I have a choice between white bread or some home-made sourdough einkorn wheat bread, I prefer to choose the latter. But, also, sometimes we don't have options. You might either have to have the processed bread or no food at all.

Most male biohackers would tell you that you should skip the meal instead and fast. But, as a woman, I know that may potentially start a domino effect of obsessing about the next meal, orthorexia, or "refeeding syndrome," when you overeat on your next meal to make up for the one you missed. I always prefer real food, no question about it. But if it's not available, I simply adjust. I'll eat in the right order, have some ACV, and move on with my life. I don't exist to work for food; food exists to work for me.

And, if I'm being perfectly honest (and I always will be with you), I don't always obey these preferences even when I *do* have a choice. But that's my point: we're not meant to. Sometimes, it's wildly inconvenient for my hosts. Sometimes, I'm in bio-slacker mode and can't feel motivated to do better. Sometimes, I just need a break from adulting and getting everything right. Sometimes (more like "every day"), people watch my stories online and say: "Aggie, how come you eat pizza? That isn't biohacking!" But to me, biohacking is being aware of all the toxins and then having free will to choose them consciously. It's being able to navigate around the various challenges like a dance. It's not about not living your life, terrified of the real world. Because that seems like a prison to me.

6 Biohacking Eating Lifestyle Preferences

1. Choose a protein-centered diet.
2. Quality above all.
3. Eat to nourish your gut.
4. Slow cook.
5. Chew your calories.
6. Eat when relaxed.

Preference 1: Macros Matter, but Protein Matters Most

Today's women don't eat enough protein because we were trained to fear proper meals; instead, we nibble (mostly on carbs). You can observe this just by sitting at a cafe for a few hours and watching what people eat. I do it all the time when I'm back home in Bali.

I remember one warm sunny day right after New Year's. All the tables outside were wooden, and one had a tree growing through the middle of it. You could almost hear the nearby ocean, an occasional scooter crossing the street, and "terima kasih," which means "thank you" in Bahasa, the local language.

The server brought out a plate of steak and eggs and a plate of waffles. He placed the steak and eggs in front of Jacob, my fiancé, and the waffles in front of me. After viewing the people around us, I guess it was a fair assumption, but in this case, he was wrong.

A blond woman is sitting at 11:00 with a friend; both are having orange juice and a smoothie bowl. There's a couple at 5:00. He's eating eggs, and she's having a smoothie. A group of girls behind me have a table laden with pancakes, waffles, smoothies, and pastries. Not a single woman appears to have ordered a savory breakfast except me. I'm not telling you this to shame anyone else's breakfast choices. But afterward, I did ask women in my community why they thought this was the case.

"I feel too manly ordering a steak on a date," one student told me. "I don't want the guy to think I eat a lot."

"I feel like if I drink my breakfast, I'm not going to put on weight," another one said.

We have already chatted about how crucial a savory breakfast is, but now I want to talk with you about the fact that it's equally important to have at least 30g of protein at every meal. But before we do, let's make sure we're on the same page.

Macro Breakdown

"Macros" is short for macronutrients, the nutrients your body needs in large amounts to get energy and keep everything running smoothly. Think of your body like a car: Proteins are the building materials to make and repair the car, carbs are the gasoline that keeps it running, and fats are like the oil that keeps everything functioning smoothly. And just like a car, you need the right balance to keep everything in good shape!

Proteins
These are like the body's building blocks. They help repair and build tissues, like muscle, skin, and hair. They also make enzymes, hormones, and other body chemicals.

Carbohydrates

Carbs are your body's main fuel source. They break down into glucose, which gives you the energy to do everything from breathing to lifting weights.

Fats

Fats are a rich energy source and are essential for supporting cell growth, protecting your organs, and keeping your body warm. They also help your body absorb some nutrients and produce vital hormones.

Your macro breakdown will change based on what part of your cycle you're in, which I'll share in an upcoming chapter, but I want you to understand the principles first.

Protein

I am a big fan of a protein-centered diet, even though some male biohackers would insist you need to do keto to get the most benefits. When we get more advanced, we will focus on a fat-centered diet in the first phase of our cycle, but I don't want to overwhelm you right now.

In general, women don't eat enough protein, and I have a feeling you might be one of those women. Protein keeps you full longer and grows your muscle—but it's not like the Gold's Gym bodybuilder mascot. (*Random side note:* I used to see Arnold Schwarzenegger there daily when I was a member. It simultaneously made me feel like I was a *very serious weight lifter* and also like I was just playing around on a movie set because, I mean, come on. I'm lifting mere feet away from the Terminator himself?! That can't be real.)

Muscle storage matters because muscles are better for storing insulin. Dr Gabrielle Lyon, a muscle expert, recommends 1.6 grams/kilogram or 1 gram/pound ideal body weight daily and 30g of protein three times a day at each meal for a total of 90g per day.

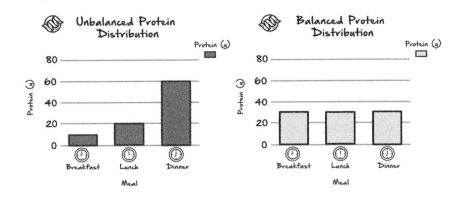

It's common in the U.S. to have a low-protein breakfast, a light lunch, and a high-protein dinner. As women, however, we need to be more deliberate about eating protein with every meal, making sure we hit 30 grams at each meal to stimulate muscle protein synthesis (which keeps the fat in your body that keeps you from wrinkling and looking older than you are).

On top of that, when your protein intake is low, carbs and fats are likely unbalanced, causing your body to store more fat and causing your blood sugar to be negatively affected. The more protein you eat, the more muscle you have; the more muscle you have, the more insulin receptors you have, and the better you manage glucose spikes.

This also means you crave fewer sugary foods and have fewer energy crushes and more balanced hormones. It's a win-win. Remember, fill up on protein first and then eat carbs and sugars (fructose) after protein and fats, and only if you still have room.

My protein preferences are grass-fed steak, pasture-raised eggs, lamb, venison, wild-caught fish, pork, and free-range pasture-raised poultry. (Some biohackers are against poultry, but I personally think it's hard to live without it. As usual, it's your call!)

Fat

I feel bad for fat. Fat has been misunderstood for years and needs a better marketing team to help people understand that fat doesn't make you fat, sugar does! Crazy, right? Fat is often demonized as the nutrient that causes weight gain, but this is simply not true. In reality, fats are a superfood—they're crucial for brain health, nutrient absorption, and hormone production, especially in women.

Dietary fat doesn't directly translate into body fat, rather, it's an essential source of energy and is critical for the absorption of vitamins A, D, E, and K. Women's bodies rely on fat for reproductive health, as fats are the building blocks for hormone production and regulation, including key hormones like estrogen and progesterone.

Plus, fats can help with weight management because they provide a sense of fullness after meals, which can reduce overall calorie intake by curbing overeating. Remember, it's the type and amount of fat that matters—avoid seed oils, trans fats, and partially hydrogenated oils.

My fat preferences include coconut oil, grass-fed butter and ghee, MCT oil, olive oil, avocado oil, and coconut milk.

Carbs

Carbohydrates, often vilified, are far more complex and critical to our well-being than we're led to believe, especially for women. We rely on carbohydrates for the maintenance of hormonal balance; diets consistently low in carbs, such as a strict ketogenic regimen, can disrupt the production of essential hormones like progesterone, potentially leading to irregular menstrual cycles. That's why we will adjust our carb intake throughout the month.

The key lies in the type of carbohydrates consumed. Nature has provided us with nutrient-dense, complex carbs found in fruits, vegetables, and legumes. These natural carbohydrates come bundled with vitamins, minerals, and dietary fiber, which are integral to gut health, satiety, and sustained energy release.

On the flip side, the modern diet is flooded with "man-made," simple carbohydrates. These are typically stripped of their nutritional value and fiber during processing and include white bread, pastries, sugary drinks, and other ultra-processed foods. Such carbs lead to rapid spikes in blood sugar and insulin levels, contributing to a roller coaster of energy highs and lows and a host of long-term health issues when consumed excessively.

The science is clear: quality and context matter when it comes to carbohydrate intake.

Nature made both starchy and non-starchy, and the beautiful thing is that you can choose from both kinds! Feel free to eat as much as you like from this list of my preferences. Non-starchy preferences include zucchini, cucumbers, asparagus, celery, mushrooms, cabbage, broccoli, cauliflower, Brussels sprouts, sprouts, arugula, and lettuce. Starchy preferences include pumpkin, butternut squash, carrot, arrowroot, sweet potato, and yams.

Sugar

Sugar sneaks its way into our diets far beyond the occasional dessert, hiding in many everyday foods where we least expect it, like bread, condiments (such as ketchup and BBQ sauce), milk alternatives, energy drinks, and even "healthy" salad dressings. These unexpected sources can quickly accumulate, making it all too easy to surpass the recommended daily sugar intake without realizing it.

In the U.S., it's a particularly pervasive problem, with the average American consuming about 77 grams of sugar daily—*triple* the advised limit for women. While treating yourself to a sweet treat now and then is perfectly fine, the real issue lies in the hidden sugars that sneak into your food and contribute to excessive fructose consumption, leading to various health issues when ingested in large quantities over time.

Biohacking recommends no more than 25g of fructose a day, roughly 3.5 cups of berries, about two medium-sized apples, or two large bananas. It's easy to top that threshold with as little as half a can of soda or a single sweetened latte. I know some of you are wondering if you should use artificial sweeteners to help keep these numbers a bit lower.

In a word, NO. In three words: NO! NO! NO! In ten words: NO! NO! NO! NO! NO! NO! NO! NO! NO! NO! Please don't. Splenda (sucralose) and aspartame are both artificial sweeteners, and while they may *sound* better with your glucose in view, they are so much worse for your health.

There is a tremendous amount of evidence linking artificial sweeteners to an increased risk of metabolic disorders, such as obesity and metabolic syndrome or insulin resistance (not to mention other conditions like cancer). Many of those studies suggest that consuming these intensely sweet, calorie-free artificial sweeteners may increase cravings for sweet foods and beverages, potentially leading to overeating and weight gain.

Preference 2: Choose Nature-Made Food Over Man-Made and Quality Above All

I would love for you to become a qualitarian—someone who may or may not follow a specific dietary plan but who always evaluates the quality of food before consuming it.

The term was coined by Dr. Mark Hyman when he said: "I'm a *qualitarian* who focuses on eating unprocessed, fresh, whole foods that are—when possible—organic and locally grown or raised."

A biohacker focused on quality asks questions like:

- Where did this food come from?
- Are the ingredients naturally sourced?
- If it's animal-based, was the animal treated well? Did it have access to the sun and grass? Was the animal happy and relatively free?
- Will it nourish me or create inflammation in my body?

High-quality food is clean, dense in nutrients, and benefits our bodies. I'm talking about fruits and vegetables that are free from chemicals and sourced as locally as feasible, as longer gaps between harvest and consumption result in decreased nutrient content.

Look for meat and eggs from happy animals, free from hormones, antibiotics, and other growth-stimulating injections. Seek out foods that are not genetically modified (that means you'll probably avoid most soy, corn, oats, and wheat) and avoid those that contain heavy metals (like many fish) or anti-nutrients.

The goal of your diet is to nourish your body—or, at the very least, not make you sick.

Whenever you can, prioritize foods that are pasture-raised, raw, unpasteurized, unhomogenized, unprocessed, fresh, not frozen (or defrosted), grass-fed, organic, free from hormones, free from antibiotics, free from other growth-stimulating injections, from a rich soil that hasn't been depleted from herbicides and overfarming (aim for regenerative farms), and heirloom or locally seasonal.

These types of food can get very expensive very fast—especially at large chain stores that claim to cater to these types of products. But between your local farmer's market and Costco, you will probably be surprised to find some really good quality ingredients that won't cost you an arm and a leg.

Weston A. Price

A lot of people think I started eating meat because of pressure from my meat-eating fiancé or because I got obsessed with Dave Asprey's work, but the truth is, I started eating meat because of Weston A. Price and his work. I mean, the other two are also true; Asprey is an inspiration, and my fiancé is *so damn cute*. But mostly the Weston A. Price thing.

Weston A. Price was the OG biohacker—a Canadian dentist in the 1920s who couldn't believe the tooth decay in even his youngest patients. He thought, *Hang on, it doesn't seem right that I even have a job in the first place. Dentists or orthodontics shouldn't exist. Nature wouldn't create us to need a dentist.*

Yet, tooth decay was such a serious issue even in the 1920s that suicides from toothaches were not unheard of. Something felt fishy to Dr. Price, so he traveled around the world to see if dental rot starting in childhood was showing up elsewhere. He suspected diet had something to do with it, so one of his goals as he embarked on his journey was to find the perfect one.

He first went to a remote village in Switzerland, accessible only via hiking paths. Their diet included cheese, milk, and sourdough bread. (*Wait, Aggie, aren't these the things you are about to tell me not to eat? Where were the Swiss chard smoothies? That would seem apt, given their location.* Sit tight. We're going to talk about that.)

What did he find? Zero cavities and perfectly straight teeth in all the children. He was also struck by their high cheekbones. He wrote that he "never witnessed a baby crying," and women gave birth to babies "with great ease, often at night with their husband next to them, fast asleep." Um … are you thinking that this sounds like a science fiction book? Because it sure does to me. However, Dr. Price's findings offered a fascinating hypothesis.

He believed that poor diet caused the bone structures to be under-developed, making many women's pelvic openings narrow and oval rather than round. And that's a very difficult shape for the baby's head to get out. That, he speculated, was why childbirth had become so difficult, so painful, and often life-threatening for a lot of women.

Visiting that remote village and many others ranging from the Arctic Circle to the Amazon rainforests to remote Pacific islands over the next decade introduced him to some of the healthiest teeth and humans he'd ever seen. He was trying to find a common theme between all these native cultures, and here is what he concluded.

There is no perfect diet. The diet in each group was very different, but they all had a few things in common: none were fully vegan, and none were eating mass-produced, processed foods (which were already an issue even in the 1920s). They lived off the land, avoided lean meat, and prioritized fat and organ meat, as well as fermented and pickled food. We *need* a little animal protein, but depending on where you live, it doesn't have to be much.

Based on his research, Dr. Price documented almost 100 years ago what biohacking and science have "discovered" much more recently: processed foods, seed oils, and diets that are too far separated from the source of the food are the reason we are struggling with poor health today.

You aren't just what you eat—you are also *what your food ate*. Grass-fed and pasture-raised meat comes from animals allowed to graze on natural grasses and plants throughout their lives, as opposed to being raised in confined feedlots and fed a diet primarily consisting of grain. Organic and heirloom vegetables have higher nutritional values because they aren't being forced to grow from depleted soil or genetically modified seeds.

Does it mean you can't be vegan as a biohacker? Girl, if a cauliflower can be pizza, you, too, can be anything you want! But as someone who has been vegan and who knows a lot of ex-vegan-turned-biohackers, adding a little ethically raised meat occasionally will make a lot of health issues easier.

Even better? Try incorporating a "whole animal" approach by using nutrient-dense organ meat like liver, spleen, stomach, and even the brain, and use the marrow or make beef bone broth to get more calcium (there are recipes on the website.)

These are great for women who are trying to get pregnant, not to mention eating the whole animal is a more sustainable and respectful approach to meat consumption. It reduces waste and ensures that the animal's sacrifice provides maximum nourishment.

Bursting the Vegan Bubble—the Circle of Life

My students often ask me if it's okay to be vegan on the biohacking eating lifestyle. As someone who was vegan for almost eight years, I totally understand this question. Being vegan was my identity. I felt so good (and sometimes better than others or judgemental of them) when I knew that my lifestyle and diet choices didn't contribute to the suffering of animals. Over the course of seven years, however, I slowly but surely felt more dependent on coffee, snacking, napping, and "pushing through" the day instead of feeling like there was unlimited energy overflowing from me—how I often feel now. But I didn't want to give up being vegan and become an "animal killer" or contribute to the horrible treatment in meat factories. No way, no how. Over my dead body.

Well, that was a bit of an ironic statement because my body was having a harder and harder time staying healthy. When I heard

Dave Asprey talk on his podcast about the importance of grass-fed meat, I wanted so badly for him to be wrong. But then he shared a story of visiting a Buddhist monastery in Laos, where they not only drank tea with yak butter, they also ate meat. When he challenged them, they said, "One death, many dinners."

The difference is that if you are a vegan, you actually may end up killing more animals per meal than a carnivore because of collateral damage. A carnivore only takes one life with its dinner, meanwhile, there are dozens of rabbits, foxes, mice, insects, birds, worms, and more that are killed in the process of harvesting soy, wheat, and corn. When you look at the death-per-meal ratio, there are many more lives taken when producing items that are meat replacements than in the butchering of a single animal for human consumption.

As much as I wanted (and still want) to separate myself from any kind of animal cruelty, no human is completely removed from animal death. This is something that the Biohacking Eating Lifestyle and the vegan diet have in common: We have a deep reverence for animals, and we do not support cruel factory farms. Small, regenerative farming, where there is deep gratitude and respect for the animal's life, is one of the core principles of responsible consumption in this kind of biohacking.

Eat Locally

Bestie, repeat after me: *Celebrate your seasons and infradian rhythm.* In our male-centered world, everything is available everywhere all the time, and the year's natural waning and waxing means very little. But if you step into your feminine energy, you will fall in love with seasons, with the impermanence of spring and summer, and you will start celebrating them by eating seasonally. Fruits and vegetables can have a higher nutrient content when harvested during their natural growing season.

For example, a study in the *Journal of Agricultural and Food Chemistry* showed that vitamin C content in broccoli was twice as high when harvested in the fall than in the spring, which follows broccoli's natural pattern. Seasonal produce also tends to be fresher, as it hasn't been stored as long or transported as far, leading to better taste and texture.

Eating seasonally often means eating locally. Foods grown out of season may require more chemical assistance in terms of pesticides and herbicides. Seasonal foods are usually more abundant and thus often less expensive than out-of-season foods that have been shipped in from somewhere else.

The Biohacking Eating Lifestyle prioritizes locally sourced and seasonal foods, which support the body's needs throughout the year. (Many diet plans do this, too. I'm not claiming to be totally original here.) Locally grown produce in farmers' markets traveled an average distance of 27 miles to reach you, compared to the 1,500 miles traveled by conventionally sourced produce (The Center for Urban Education about Sustainable Agriculture (CUESA) conducted a study in 2010).

As fruits and vegetables are allowed to mature naturally, they develop a broader range of vitamins, minerals, and antioxidants that contribute to optimal health. On the other hand, imported produce is harvested prematurely to compensate for the travel time, which means it hasn't had a chance to maximize its growth. Choosing local produce reduces the carbon footprint associated with food transportation, as well. This helps sustain local agriculture, preserves farmland, and creates job opportunities in the community.

Heirloom vegetables are a bit like cherished family treasures passed down through generations. Instead of jewelry or antique furniture, though, they're seeds! Unlike hybrid vegetables, which are the result of two different varieties being cross-pollinated to produce a new variety, heirlooms are open-pollinated, which means they are pollinated by plants of the same species, resulting in seeds that are almost identical to seeds from 50, 100, or even more years back. Many believe heirloom vegetables taste better, offering richer and more complex flavors.

At the grocery store, we look for the biggest, smoothest, blemish-free vegetables and leave the ugly ones behind like an ugly duckling. Interestingly, vegetable blemishes or imperfections can result from environmental stressors, like insect nibbling or exposure to the elements. When plants face these challenges, they often produce phytochemicals to protect themselves.

It just so happens that our gut *loves* natural phytochemicals. So, a vegetable with more stress might be packed with more of these amazing nutrients. Small-scale farmers or organic farms that are more likely to produce "imperfect" veggies might also be using farming practices that prioritize soil health over the cosmetic appearance of their plants. Healthy soil contains a wider variety of beneficial microbes and minerals, which can be incorporated into the vegetables during the growing process, making them more nutrient-dense than their corporate mega-farm cousins.

Preference 3: Feed Your Gut

We share 99.9% of our DNA with other humans but only 10% of our gut. We probably all know someone who can eat whatever they want, not gain weight, and have a flat stomach. But don't envy them—envy their gut!

Want to know another fun fact? You can look at someone's gut bacteria and tell if they are obese or skinny. Even crazier? You can transplant poop that belongs to a skinny person into the rectum of an obese one, and *they will lose weight*! (It's called fecal matter transplant, and it's a booming business, however, it's not yet available in the U.S.)

All of that to say, your gut is a serious business—and women's gut biomes are even more important than men's! We inherit our gut from our mothers and pass on our microbiome to our children, so if you don't have a strong gut, it could be that your mom didn't either.

Now you can see why I love and prioritize my gut so much! A healthy gut is vital to your overall mental and physical well-being. It connects to your digestion and nutrient absorption, immune system, inflammation, weight balance, hormones, and even mood and brain function. Whether you are sick or healthy, pay attention to your gut to achieve the radiant health you deserve.

In fact, I love my gut so much, let's dive into gut health itself.

What Is Your Gut?

Imagine your gut is like New York City.

NYC is home to millions of people from all over the world, each playing their unique role, much like your microbiome is home to trillions of bacteria, viruses, fungi, and other microorganisms co-existing. There are some good guys and some bad ones, but as long as the good guys are in the majority, the city is in control and thriving.

Walk the streets of NYC, and you'll hear languages from all over the world. Similarly, the microbiome is incredibly diverse, with thousands of species coexisting, each contributing its own "skills" and "talents" to the community.

Every individual in NYC has a role, from taxi drivers zipping people across town to chefs preparing your next UberEats order to women in suits killing it in finance. Similarly, in the microbiome, each bacterium has a job. Some break down fiber, others produce essential vitamins, and some even help fend off harmful invaders.

And just like NYC needs balance, the microbiome needs balance, too. An overgrowth of certain bacteria in your gut is like when, say, rats start to overrun the city. Similarly, factors like diet, medications (like antibiotics), and stress can shift and shape the microbiome, changing its landscape and its vibe.

Yet despite challenges, NYC always seems to bounce back, always evolving and adapting—just like the microbiome. When given the right "resources" (prebiotics, probiotics, and a healthy diet), it can recover and flourish after disruptions.

If your gut is healthy, it should be filled with trillions of different bacteria, mostly good. If you're dealing with digestive woes like bloating, gas, or irregular bowel movements, however, your gut might be distressed. Suddenly, finding you can't stomach foods that never bothered you before, such as dairy or nuts, is another hint that your gut health needs attention. Even persistent fatigue and mood swings can often be traced back to gut issues because of how well you absorb nutrients.

Your skin mirrors your internal health, too; flare-ups like acne or eczema could point to a gut imbalance. I discovered this when my skin improved as I healed my gut. Unexplained weight changes and frequent colds are additional clues that your gut might be out of whack and contributing to metabolic imbalances and a weakened immune system. Finally, if you're constantly battling inflammation or unexplained aches, it's worth considering whether—you guessed it—your gut health might be a potential contributor.

What Damages Your Gut?

Okay, so you're clued in on why gut health is crucial. But what are the main villains wreaking havoc on it? (*Are we still doing the NYC thing? I was going to turn this into a superhero metaphor. No? Is it played out? Okay. Fine. I get it. No, no. I'm not mad—just disappointed. ANY-WAY.*) Topping the list is an unhealthy diet—too much processed food, refined sugars, bad fats like seed oils, and not enough fiber can throw off your gut bacteria and inflame your intestines. Snacking nonstop doesn't give your gut a break to reset, either. Then there's antibiotics; they're like dropping a bomb in a lush Costa Rican jungle, decimating not just the bad but also the good bacteria in your gut, making recovery tough. Antibiotics are lifesavers but should be a last resort, not the first line of defense.

Chronic stress messes with your gut, too, tweaking gut motility and bacterial balance—it's why taming my stress helped calm my IBS symptoms. Don't forget infections and parasites; these unwanted guests can damage your gut's lining and function. Popping NSAIDs frequently? They could be irritating your stomach, upping your ulcer and gastritis risk. And, yes, excessive alcohol does a number on your digestive tract—so go easy on those porn star martinis.

If certain foods trigger inflammation for you, like gluten or lactose, they're not your gut's friends. Autoimmune diseases, such as Crohn's or celiac, can also attack and inflame your gut. And it's not just what you ingest; environmental toxins like pesticides and heavy metals are gut health foes, too. Lastly, don't underestimate the power of sleep; without enough shut-eye, your gut can get out of sync. All these factors can chip away at your gut health, so keep them in check for your overall well-being.

How to Feed Your Gut

Since there are such great benefits to having a healthy gut, including weight loss, reduced inflammation, better insulin resistance, reduced allergies and infections, a bioavailability of nutrients, and better overall health, let's take a careful look into how you can accomplish this.

First off, eat the rainbow! Try to consume at least 50 different plants a week (and 30 grams of fiber a day).

Some microbes are like picky eaters: they thrive and grow on certain foods and die off when you don't eat enough of their favorite foods. The more diverse the diet, the more diverse the microbiome. Fifty plants a week comes out to 200 a month. I know that may sound wild to you since the average woman in the U.S. eats a fraction of that—75% of the world's food supply comes from 12 plants and five animals—but there are so many options that can make diversifying your intake fun and delicious. You can even include fermented foods like sauerkraut, kefir, and kimchi, which are rich in beneficial probiotics that support gut health.

Other Tips to Support Your Gut:

- Cutting down on sugar can starve out the bad bacteria in your gut, so dialing it back can lead to a healthier microbiome.

- Make sure to chew your food thoroughly to aid digestion and feed good bacteria.

- Hydration is essential—it helps keep everything moving smoothly.

- Consider a gentle detox to reduce inflammation and give your gut a break.

- Apple cider vinegar can be a game changer for stomach acid because of the ways that it boosts digestion.

- Probiotics from supplements or fermented foods like yogurt and kimchi are your gut's allies, as are polyphenol-rich foods like berries, dark chocolate, and flaxseeds.

- Try to go organic to avoid gut-harming pesticides, and embrace intermittent fasting to let your digestive system reset.

- Don't forget the surprising benefits of having a pet, getting your hands dirty, and soaking up some vitamin D outside. These activities not only expose you to beneficial microbes but also help manage stress—another win for gut health. So get out, get active, and let nature be your gut's best friend.

Preference 4: Slow Cooking

In biohacking, it's not just about the quality of your food but also about how you prepare it. You could source the finest grass-fed steak, but if it's charred to a crisp, you aren't going to get any nutritional benefits from it. It's like my grandma used to say: Good food takes time. She'd work magic with a slow cooker, turning a simple chicken leg into a tender delight over gentle heat. But today, with the rush of modern life, slow cooking seems like a luxury. We're geared up for quick fixes, and, in turn, we are missing out on the healthiest cooking methods.

We should focus on gentle cooking; try steaming veggies *al dente*, baking meats at low temperatures, slow-cooking stews, simmering broths, poaching eggs, and grilling lightly or using *sous vide* and pressure cookers.

On the flip side, it's wise to steer clear of anything fried, broiled, barbecued, stir-fried, burnt, blackened, charred, deep-fried, or microwaved. High heat can oxidize fats, creating harmful free radicals and forming Advanced Glycation End Products (AGEs), which are nasty compounds that can accelerate aging from the inside out.

Preference 5: Chew Your Calories Rather Than Drink Them

Not too long ago, the pre-biohacking, mainstream Aggie barely ever chewed her food. I started my day with a latte, celery juice, and a smoothie, followed by avocado toast and maybe another smoothie and a matcha. Even though smoothies are healthy, I ended up bloated and baffled.

Drinking your calories, whether it's fruit juices, smoothies, or alcohol, often doesn't provide the same fullness as eating whole foods. Research shows that calories consumed in liquid form aren't as satisfying as those consumed in solid food. This means you might consume more overall calories throughout the day as your body struggles to feel sated (especially when you drink through a straw and bypass the tongue).

While 100% fruit juices and smoothies provide some vitamins and minerals, they lack the fiber in the whole fruit. Fiber helps to slow digestion, keeps you full, and stabilizes your blood sugar levels. Smoothies that are made with banana, when drunk, hit your digestive system much faster, leading to a massive glucose spike.

On top of that, portion control is more challenging. It can be difficult to control portions when you're drinking your calories. A couple of gulps could be equivalent to a whole meal's calories, but it won't fill you up like a meal would. Research has suggested that drinking your calories can lead to increased insulin resistance and inflammation, which can negatively impact your metabolism.

Additionally, a study in the *Journal of the American Dietetic Association* found that when people consumed a meal with a caloric beverage, they ate roughly the same amount of food as when they consumed a meal with a non-caloric drink, leading to an increase in total calorie intake.

In one of my favorite books, *Breath: The New Science of a Lost Art*, author James Nestor emphasizes the importance of chewing. Remember when I mentioned that Weston Price noticed that the groups with the healthiest diets generally had healthy ancestors with high cheekbones and straight teeth? He theorized that they ate tougher, raw foods that required significant chewing. This consistent workout helped to develop their facial bones and muscles.

Our modern diet of soft, processed foods like smoothies and pasta, which require very little chewing, might contribute to crooked teeth and even more restricted airways. In his book, Nestor looks at the connection between chewing and breathing. Strong, well-developed chewing muscles can help keep the airway and your soft palate open, potentially leading to better, healthier breathing. (We will look at why breathing is the ultimate biohack in a later chapter.)

Chewing activates the production of saliva, which not only aids digestion but also helps keep the mouth clean, reduces acid reflux, and can even boost concentration and memory.

So what do I do when I'm listening to my body, and it is very politely asking for a smoothie to meet some nutritional need?

- I make or ask for my smoothies to be very thick, almost like smoothie bowls, and eat them with a spoon. I hold the smoothie in my mouth before swallowing to activate the digestive enzymes.
- I opt for keto-style smoothies that don't include added sugar (like honey) or very sweet fruit like banana, pineapple, or mango to avoid a massive glucose spike.
- I always add protein to them (either collagen protein or Biohacking Bestie Busy Bee Vanilla Protein).
- I have healthy chewing gum afterward to activate my stomach acid.
- I don't have them every day. (I like chewing my food! A sturdier texture is more satisfying to me in addition to the health benefits of chewing.)

Preference 6: Eat When Relaxed

I used to be the queen of speed-eating, multitasking through meals with one eye on my phone and the other on a video of some lifestyle guru somewhere who always seemed to be so much more put together than I could ever hope to be. Eating was just another box to tick off in my daily to-dos. But with that pace came unwanted bloating and indigestion.

And it turns out, the struggle was more than just physical—my vagus nerve was struggling too. The vagus nerve is a fascinating part of our body. It's the longest nerve we have, extending from the brain down through the neck and into the belly. It's like a two-way communication superhighway between the brain and the gut, transmitting signals in both directions. Think of it as a biological telephone wire that helps control and relay information among various organs, including the heart, lungs, and digestive tract.

But why does it matter, especially when it comes to mindful eating? The vagus nerve is a key player in the parasympathetic nervous system—the part of your nervous system that tells your body to "rest and digest." It helps regulate many functions you don't consciously control, like heart rate and digestive processes.

When you practice mindful eating, you're giving your vagus nerve a workout. By eating slowly, savoring each bite, and paying attention to your food, you activate this nerve, which helps improve digestion and signals fullness to your brain. It also helps to manage stress by promoting a more relaxed state, which is optimal for digestion and overall well-being.

In other words, by being mindful of what and how you eat, you're tuning into and toning your vagus nerve, which can lead to better digestion, a sense of calm, and a more harmonious dialogue between your gut and your brain. It's like sending a "calm down, everything's okay" message throughout your body, which is priceless in today's fast-paced world.

I've come to realize the power of pausing in the "rest and digest" mode, or as I prefer to say, "rest and receive." There's a profound lesson here, especially for us as women, to accept abundance without the reflex to reciprocate instantly—to embrace our worthiness of simply receiving. It's a tough lesson, going against the instinct to immediately ask, "What can I do for you?" or "How can I pay it back?" But it's essential for sinking into our feminine energy and unlocking true relaxation.

Mindful Eating Tips

Activating your vagus nerve and practicing mindful eating can enhance your digestive health and overall well-being. Cold exposure stimulates your vagus nerve, so briefly splashing your face with cold water, holding an ice cube in your hand, or simply taking off a layer of clothing before a meal can activate the vagus nerve.

Gargling water or humming during cooking or before eating can stimulate the vagus nerve since it runs right behind the throat.

In the state of fight or flight, our bodies are on high alert; our pupils contract, granting us a sort of tunnel vision. Research suggests that by consciously directing our eyes to look left, right, up, and down, we can nudge our bodies out of this heightened state and into a calmer "rest and digest" mode. (As opposed to up-up-down-down-left-right-left-right-B-A, which will power you up for a 1980s Nintendo game.) As we relax, our pupils dilate back to a state of rest, broadening our field of vision to fully engage with our surroundings.

Finally, start your meal by taking several deep breaths. Deep, diaphragmatic breathing stimulates the vagus nerve and can help shift your body into a calm state. Take a moment before eating to express gratitude for your food. This practice can help shift your focus and awareness. Chew each bite thoroughly, and put down your knife and fork between bites. Slowing down helps your body better digest and absorb nutrients, giving your brain time to recognize when you're full. Pay attention to your food's smell, taste, texture, and colors. Noticing these details can enrich the eating experience and help you be more present at the meal and in the moment.

KEY TAKEAWAYS

- Embrace learning about macronutrients, toxins, and more in Level 2 of your biohacking journey. It's like going from classroom Italian to ordering in Rome—challenging but enriching. Remember, there's no shame in revisiting the basics if you feel overwhelmed.

- Prefer but don't obsess about a protein-centered diet and become a "qualitarian," focusing on high-quality, nutrient-dense foods. This approach involves selecting unprocessed, organic, and locally sourced foods and understanding the impact of what you eat on your body.

- Include animal proteins in your diet, however small, especially ethically raised meat and the health benefits of a balanced diet.

- Your gut is like a bustling New York City, with its diverse microbiome playing a crucial role in overall health. A healthy gut impacts everything from digestion and mood to hormone balance and immune function.

- Eat the rainbow and practice mindful eating. This includes chewing your calories instead of drinking them, enjoying a variety of foods to nourish the gut, and embracing the art of slow cooking to preserve nutritional value.

- Eat in a relaxed state to activate the parasympathetic nervous system, using techniques like deep breathing before meals, cold exposure to stimulate the vagus nerve, and taking time to savor and appreciate food, enhancing digestion and overall well-being.

CHAPTER 5

WHAT NOT TO EAT

"There's nothing wrong with you. You're just a sensitive soul living in a sick society. If you feel like you don't belong in this world, it's because you were born to help create a better one."

–Lalah Delia

Avoid Toxins and Anti-Nutrients

"Society is eating so much junk food that eating real food is called 'dieting.'"

–Unknown

In the previous chapter, we focused on what to eat; now it's time to focus on what to avoid *preferably*. (There's that word again. Remember, there's no shame here. It's about doing your best and moving forward.)

In today's society, we are surrounded by food, chemicals, and toxins that are often the root cause of all diseases. However, modern medicine focuses on the symptoms, not the root cause.

Acne is a perfect example of this! The go-to solutions are often top-ical treatments like benzoyl peroxide or salicylic acid, or in more severe cases, prescription medications like Accutane. While these treatments can effectively reduce or eliminate the visible symptoms (pimples, blackheads, etc.), they don't always address what's *causing* the acne in the first place.

Acne can be triggered by different factors, many of which are inter-nal. Hormonal imbalances, poor gut health, food sensitivities (like dairy, gluten, or anti-nutrients), and even stress can all be root causes of acne. So, while you might be able to clear up your skin tempo-rarily with topical treatments, if you don't address the underlying issue, those breakouts will probably make a comeback.

There are a lot of foods that can cause inflammation in your body. Have you ever woken up swollen with puffy eyes, rings that are too tight, or feeling like you're carrying an extra cushion of water around your hips? That's inflammation. But even blisters, brain fog, or a lack of focus can be signs. In biohacking, we try to lower inflam-mation as much as possible because it can cause or exacerbate many diseases.

Inflammation is the body's natural response to pathogens, toxins, stress, or trauma. For example, when you cut yourself, your body feels the injury, swells, and signals the brain that it needs to heal this cut. This is known as acute inflammation.

Chronic inflammation, however, can be caused by eating foods that cause inflammation in the body, placing our bodies in a con-stant state of "healing." This sounds good—I mean, we all want to heal, right? But attempting to do so for years on end without a break will wear the body out. Wouldn't it be better to *be healed* than constantly *trying* to heal? The solution is to eat anti-inflammatory foods instead.

Inflammation can mess with your metabolism, lead to unexpected weight gain, and cause issues like bloating, gas, or even more severe symptoms. Chronic inflammation can give you sore muscles and sap your energy, making you feel tired more easily.

In this chapter, I want to share with you many of the foods known to trigger inflammation in your body. This is not meant to scare you (although some feelings of "What the hell?" are normal and welcomed).

I'll explain what these foods are and show you how to not only avoid them, but also how to help your body naturally remove them from your system, hence removing the root cause of some of the potential issues you might be dealing with.

Obesogens

Obesogens are chemicals that confuse the hell out of your hormones and body. They make you store extra fat, screw up your metabolism, and literally cause obesity (hence the name. I know. Not very creative, but oh-so-telling). Obesogens can increase the number and size of fat cells by boosting the body's fat-storage capacity; remember, we love our fat—but we love it as nature intended it, not boosted by artificial means. These chemicals alter the way the body regulates feelings of hunger and fullness, which can lead to overeating and shift how the body metabolizes calories, so instead of using the energy efficiently, the body stores more of it as fat.

What are some examples?

- pesticides (such as glyphosate, yet again!)
- plastics with BPA
- high fructose corn syrup
- sugar substitutes such as NutraSweet
- phthalates and perfluorooctanoic acid (PFOA)

- even some natural compounds, like those found in soy, may act as obesogens.

Places you will routinely find phthalates include:

- perfume
- lotions
- makeup
- deodorant
- shampoo
- shower curtains
- food packaging
- inflatable toys
- plastic wrap

PFOA specifically can also be found in a long list of consumer and industrial products:

- nonstick cookware coatings such as Teflon
- stain-resistant fabrics in carpeting, upholstery, and outdoor gear
- cleaning products such as carpet cleaners and spot removers

Seed Oils

So how did we start using seed oils? It was all thanks to a few businessmen in America in the 19th century. In the mid-1800s, the U.S. fashion industry was left with a byproduct from producing cotton—cottonseed oil. Manufacturers looked at all this resulting from their already *deeply* problematic industry (to say the least) and tried to figure out something to do with it.

Finally, after several decades of experimentation and various fruitless efforts, in 1911, Procter & Gamble realized that through a very intense hydrogenation process, cottonseed oil could be used as soap—and, even better, it could also be sold as "new lard." They came out with a new product marketed as "crystallized cottonseed oil" or Crisco.

A year later, the first instance of a heart attack was documented in medical journals. Now, I know that correlation is not causation, but the timing certainly is interesting as physicians were becoming increasingly aware of the ways that heart health was impacted by environmental factors.

In fact, in 1924, the American Heart Association (AHA) was founded as the field of cardiology became a medical specialty. Then, in 1961, the AHA came out with what they claimed was the answer to heart disease—after a massive donation by Procter & Gamble to the tune of $1.7 million (about $17.5 million adjusted for inflation).

And just what was the AHA's *totally unbiased (cough, cough)* recommendation? They suggested that everyone replace saturated fats like tallow, butter, and lard, which our ancestors ate for thousands of years, with polyunsaturated fats like those found in vegetable oils such as Crisco "to prevent heart attack and stroke."

Gee, Aggie—it must be tough working out while wearing a tinfoil hat. Okay, I hear you; that's enough conspiracy theory talk for today. But if you have the time and inclination to read up more on this topic, it's pretty fascinating—and depressing. But that's not the point of this chapter. The point is that seed oils are harmful, and you should avoid them, so let's focus on that.

Why Avoid Seed Oils?

Seed oils are a big deal because they make us sick and fat. They age us at a crazy rate, cause our skin to wrinkle, and are often the root cause of many conditions you probably struggle with.

The most commonly used seed oils in Western diets include:

- Corn oil
- Grapeseed oil
- Canola oil (also called rapeseed oil)
- Soy oil
- Sunflower oil
- Shortening
- Safflower oil
- Rice bran oil
- Cottonseed oil

They look innocent, don't they? I mean, rice bran oil? Sunflower oil? They sound so natural and lovely. Surely, this is something you want more of in your diet, right? *Nope.*

Seed oils are not stable, which means they oxidize. Oxidizing is literally the same process as rusting, but instead of on a piece of metal, it happens inside your body. The process creates free radicals (trouble-makers that damage your cells), which make you age prematurely, as well as cause wrinkles and inflammation.

Unfortunately, they are everywhere. Almost every packaged and processed food is full of vegetable oils. I'm not talking only chips, crisps, and fries; even the seemingly healthy alternatives like vegan cheese, burgers, and plant-based milks incorporate them.

Why? Well, for starters, they are cheap. That's why restaurants love using them. Also, they don't have much flavor, so they can do the heavy lifting of animal fats without interfering with the taste. If the barista added honey or white sugar to your coffee in the morning, you would know right away. You would have a sip and say, "Sorry, my coffee has some sugar in it. Can you remake it?"

But when the barista uses oat milk that is full of rapeseed oil, you're not going to take a sip and say, "Sorry, there is a cancer-causing, inflammation-inducing oil in my coffee. I don't want it." You would drink it and think, *Yummy, creamy, milky.* The problem, of course, is that since we can't taste the oils, we are often unaware of how much of them we consume. In fact, according to the latest studies, seed oils often make up 10% of our diet.

What to Do

And so even if you eat healthy at home, like I do, you still probably eat a lot of seed oils daily because they are so prevalent, even in high-end restaurants. And why is such an important ingredient not disclosed on menus?

Thankfully, some of my favorite restaurants in Bali now have a note on the menu saying, "We pride ourselves on using butter/ghee and coconut oil. Let us know your preference on how you'd like us to prepare your dish." I love this so much because it allows me to take back some control over my preferences when I am out and about.

I know it's frustrating to "be that person" at the restaurant. We all feel pressure to be a nice girl who doesn't ask challenging questions or make special requests because it's perceived as rude or pushy. But I already know that you treat waitstaff with respect, so why would that change when you order your food? Just keep being your kind self while you ask a few questions.

This is how we create change: by asking simple things like, "Could you let me know what kind of oil you use to prepare this dish?" In the U.S., better restaurants often ask if there are any dietary restrictions or allergies they should be aware of. Please believe me when I tell you that the inflammation seed oils create should be treated as seriously as lactose intolerance. They can wreak havoc on your body, and I don't want that for you.

Also, there is an app I highly recommend called Seed Oil Scout, which allows you to "dine fearlessly in the urban jungle." It discloses restaurants that use and don't use seed oils, which can help you make more informed choices.

Glyphosate

Glyphosate is like that toxic ex who just keeps slipping through the cracks and making its way back into our lives, no matter what we do to try to get rid of them (no, you don't get *another* chance). It's an herbicide most commonly known for its use in Monsanto's Roundup weed killer (ironically, a product now owned by Bayer, the vitamin and drug producer). Why should you care about a weed killer?

Well, glyphosate has become a popular character in the agriculture industry because it's good at its job—a little too good. It's used extensively on genetically modified (GM) crops like soy, corn, and canola which are engineered to resist its poison. This allows farmers to spray their fields with glyphosate, killing the weeds but not the crops. The result? Glyphosate residues can end up in our food and, thus, in our bodies (especially a film-like lining in our gut).

Glyphosate has the power to disrupt your gut microbiome. Just as it kills plants, it may also harm beneficial bacteria in your intestines, upsetting the delicate balance and potentially leading to health issues like a weakened immune system or digestive problems.

Some research has suggested links between glyphosate exposure and various health issues, like celiac disease, autism, and cancer, specifically non-Hodgkin (sometimes called non-Hodgkin's) lymphoma. This point hits home as my fiancé's beloved grandfather, who used to love gardening and for years sprayed "safe" glyphosate all over his plants, died suddenly from non-Hodgkin lymphoma. This form of cancer is ridiculously overrepresented in farmers, and there have been more than 100,000 lawsuits (and counting) brought against the Bayer corporation over this linkage.

How do you limit the glyphosate in your diet? Eat organic foods (since glyphosate isn't allowed in organic farming), wash and peel produce, opt for whole foods over processed ones, and avoid produce known to be treated with the chemical, such as oats. In fact, a whopping 99% of oats grown in the U.S. have been found to contain glyphosate.

Gluten

The gluten available in our foods today is drastically different from the quality that was available to our grandparents in their time. This makes me sad because I love bread, and I grew up having bread with almost every meal.

But why are so many people suddenly allergic to gluten or are gluten intolerant when we can trace our consumption of wheat back over 10,000 years? Back then, our wheat existed in a simpler form called einkorn. Over thousands of years, through selective breeding, we've changed the wheat to increase its yield, enhance its baking qualities, and make it resistant to diseases. It has undergone significant genetic modifications during this time.

Modern wheat now has many more chromosomes (42, compared to einkorn's 14), which gives us the super starch and super gluten. This increased gluten content gives us fluffier, softer, more appealing bread but also causes addictive behavior and overeating. The increased starch actually boosts blood glucose more than white sugar, and the gluten's disruption to the gut causes inflammation in many people.

Even if the wheat is grown organically, the modified genes remain the same. However, there's a bit of a plot twist: our bodies (especially our digestive systems) are actually hardcore fans of the "classic" gluten they evolved to digest. But for many, it's as if they're stuck in the past, not recognizing or appreciating this new, "modern" gluten.

The "Dirty Dozen"

A list published by the Environmental Working Group (EWG) each year identifies fruits and vegetables that are reported to have the highest level of pesticide residues (including glyphosate) due to the way they are harvested. Even if you can't afford to go organic with all your produce, these are the ones that the EWG consistently recommends buying organic if you can:

1. Strawberries

2. Spinach

3. Kale, collard and mustard greens

4. Nectarines

5. Apples

6. Grapes

7. Cherries

8. Peaches

9. Pears

10. Bell and hot peppers

11. Celery

12. Tomatoes

Mold

Mold is a type of fungus that can grow on many different types of food, including bread, cheese, fruits, and vegetables. Consuming moldy food can have several effects on health, some of which can be serious.

Most molds are harmless when ingested, but some produce harmful substances called mycotoxins. Mycotoxins can cause a variety of health problems, from mild reactions like allergic responses and digestive upset to more severe problems like immune system suppression, neurological damage, and cancer.

The general advice for mold on food is "When in doubt, throw it out." Some molds can be cut away, such as those on hard cheeses or firm fruits and vegetables, but others, particularly those on soft foods like bread or soft fruits and vegetables, can penetrate deep into the food and should not be consumed.

Coffee and nuts, like other foods, are susceptible to mold and can also become contaminated. This is particularly true if they are stored improperly or for too long. With coffee in particular, the mold issue is often associated with improperly stored green coffee beans. If the beans are kept in warm, humid conditions, mold can grow. The roasting process can kill the mold, but the mycotoxins can remain, which can then end up in your brewed coffee—and your body.

Heavy Metals

Heavy metals are most often found in fish and pesticides but can also show up in tap water. The biggest tip for avoiding heavy metals is to avoid tap water, as 85 percent of plumbing will have rust and lead. That's why biohackers always invest in their water. You will no longer hear me say, "Tap water is fine!" It's not, actually!

Heavy metals, such as elevated mercury levels, can have lots of adverse effects, including hair loss (now, do I have your attention?). If you feel that you have lethargy and brain fog, it is a good idea to test your heavy metals.

Sea bass, mackerel (king, Spanish), swordfish, Tuna (ahi, yellowfin, canned albacore), and salmon (farmed or Atlantic) all tend to be very high in mercury and are specifically warned against in pregnancy.

Fish low in mercury, however, include sardines (my favorite), salmon (fresh, wild), haddock, sole, and trout. Mahi Mahi, cod, and snapper are somewhere in the middle and should be consumed less regularly than the others, but they don't necessarily need to be avoided altogether.

Anti-Nutrients

When it comes to food, there are three essential components: energy (calories), nutrients (vitamins), and anti-nutrients. The last one might surprise you, but anti-nutrients are natural or synthetic elements that keep your body from absorbing nutrients in the food you eat.

Sadly, anti-nutrients can lead to an issue called "leaky gut," which results in elevated inflammation in the body. Another interesting fact is that your hunger may increase as you consume more anti-nutrients! This happens because your body can't get the nutrients it needs from these foods, so your brain tells your body that you are still hungry.

Different people react to anti-nutrients differently. For example, my body might be able to digest lectins (found in beans and peanuts) quite well; however, you might find you react to them.

Let's run through the most common anti-nutrients, and then we will look at how to avoid them (I won't leave you without a solution, don't worry!).

Lectins

Lectins are proteins that stick to the gut lining, creating a leaky gut. A leaky gut means there are "holes" in it that enable foods to leak into the bloodstream, causing inflammation and toxicity.

Lectins include eggplant, peppers, tomatoes, potatoes, whole grains such as quinoa and brown rice, lentils, and beans. The good news is that you can remove many of the lectins from your food simply by cooking it first. Ideally, though, aim to swap some of the foods that cause this inflammation with less inflammatory versions.

Here are some examples:

- Eat white rice instead of brown. Brown rice is full of lectins, other anti-nutrients, and arsenic. (What? It's true; all rice contains trace amounts of arsenic, a naturally occurring mineral in the soil, but brown rice contains about 80% more than white rice because the arsenic tends to concentrate in the hull, which is stripped from white rice but not brown.)
- Use sweet potatoes instead of white potatoes. Sweet potatoes do not have lectins and are better for managing blood sugar levels.
- Swap peanut butter for almond butter.

Phytic Acid

Phytic acid binds to magnesium, iron, calcium, and zinc, preventing them from absorbing nutrients.

Foods high in phytic acid include brown rice, oatmeal, wheat, barley, rye, almonds, walnuts, sesame seeds, flax seeds, sunflower seeds, beans, lentils, soybeans (including foods made from these products, like tofu and tempeh), and some plant-based oils. An easy hack is to use avocado, coconut, or olive oil instead of canola or seed oils.

Oxalates

Oxalates bind to calcium in your blood, creating crystals that can lead to kidney stones. Pressure cooking or cooking in general can get rid of oxalates, so avoid raw kale and spinach; cook them instead! Oxalates are also present in broccoli, cauliflower, chard, beets, parsley, and chocolate. Sprouting (allowing seeds to start to sprout before consuming them) can help reduce oxalates, as well as fermenting the plants, which can help to detoxify their natural defense compounds. We will discuss those later on in this chapter!

How to Remove Anti-Nutrients from Your Diet

Luckily, you don't need to stop eating vegetables with anti-nutrients altogether. Here are some of the ways to get rid of those unwelcome little twerps:

Soaking: Soaking vegetables in water can help reduce certain anti-nutrients like phytates and oxalates. For example, soaking beans and legumes overnight before cooking can reduce their phytate content. (Remember to discard the soaking water and cook the vegetables in fresh water.)

Fermentation: Fermenting vegetables can break down some anti-nutrients and enhance nutrient bioavailability. Fermented foods like sauerkraut and kimchi are good examples.

Cooking: Cooking vegetables can neutralize or reduce anti-nutrients. Heat can break down complex compounds, making nutrients more accessible. Boiling, steaming, or roasting vegetables are my go-to when eating kale and spinach.

Blanching: Blanching involves briefly boiling vegetables and then plunging them into ice-cold water. This method can reduce anti-nutrients while preserving many of the nutrients.

Sprouting: Sprouting seeds, grains, and legumes before consumption can decrease the levels of anti-nutrients. The sprouting process activates enzymes that break down the compounds.

Combine with Vitamin C: Vitamin C can enhance iron absorption and counteract the effects of certain anti-nutrients like phytates. Consider pairing iron-rich vegetables (e.g., spinach) with vitamin C-rich foods (e.g., citrus fruits) in your meals.

C-L-E-A-N B-O-D-Y Framework

Want to detoxify your body from all these scary chemicals you are bombarded with? Follow my C-L-E-A-N B-O-D-Y framework!

C: Clean Care

One of the most effective ways to support your body's detoxification is through (wait for it) *not feeding it toxins*. The cleaner your lifestyle, the less there is to detoxify from. Even beyond thinking about food, you can use apps such as Yuki that help you decode what's inside your skincare and bodycare; remember you absorb a lot more through skin than you realize.

L: Love Your Liver and Your Gut

The liver is your body's primary detoxification powerhouse, metabolizing your hormones and toxins. Castor oil packs, when placed on the liver, support the detoxification process. If you do my courses, you'll hear me repeat over and over again, "All disease begins in the gut," after the Greek healer Hippocrates. Your body disposes of estrogen through the gut, so it's crucial to have enough fiber to enable your gut and digestive system to work as efficiently as possible. If your gut is leaky, it will let the toxins escape, which will get into your bloodstream and *ta-da!* Even more inflammation.

E: Eliminate Through Exercise

Sweat it out! Any form of movement or perspiration: lifting, running, dance, hot yoga, sauna time, or even sex can help get those toxins out. Remember to wipe your sweat as you go to prevent it from getting reabsorbed through your skin—and drink water! Water is a natural elixir for detoxification. If you hand wash a T-shirt, don't you want to rinse off the water you're washing it with? Well, do the same for your body. Drinking mineral-rich water while breaking a sweat at least once a day is a powerful biohack to eliminate toxins. Staying well-hydrated aids the kidneys in flushing out waste and toxins from your system. Consider adding a squeeze of lemon to your water to boost detoxifying vitamin C.

A: Adaptogens and Supplements

Certain herbal teas like dandelion root, milk thistle, and nettle are renowned for their detoxifying properties. Incorporate these teas into your daily routine to support liver health and encourage toxin elimination. Also, you can take them in supplement form if you prefer.

N: Nutrition and No Food (Fasting)

You are what your food ate, remember? Watch out for growth hormones in your diet, especially in industrial dairy and chickens. Watch out, too, for pesticides, herbicides, and glyphosate, which can throw off your hormone balance. Choose organic whenever you can, wash your veggies, and avoid nonorganic wheat and oats (which are full of glyphosate). Care about your water like a maniac (and avoid tap water if possible to keep those heavy metals down). Fast intermittently to give your digestive system a much-needed break and allow your body to focus on detoxification and cellular repair. Try to keep your body in a state of autophagy.

B: Breathwork and Bedtime

Stress is a silent toxin that can wreak havoc on your body. Your parasympathetic state promotes detoxification. Quality sleep is essential for your body's natural detoxification and repair processes. Prioritize restorative sleep by creating a relaxing bedtime routine and optimizing your sleep environment.

O: Oil-Pulling and Dry Brushing

Tongue scraping and dry brushing are both ancient techniques that are cheap, easy, and effective.

Dry brushing involves running a natural fiber brush over your body (always sweeping toward the heart). This stimulates your lymphatic system, aiding toxin elimination. It can boost circulation, support detoxification, remove dead skin, support cell turnover, exfoliate your skin, reduce puffiness and cellulite, and boost energy.

Oil pulling (swishing coconut oil in your mouth) can draw out oral bacteria and toxins, and daily tongue scraping using a simple tongue-scraping tool is a must. Your tongue kickstarts the digestive process by sensing the flavors and sending signals to your stomach to get ready for the feast. When you keep your mouth and tongue healthy, you are setting yourself up for better health all around.

D: Detox Your Digestive Tract Daily

Friend, it's time to give a shit about your shit.

Let's get *reeeaaal* personal for a minute. I used to think going to the bathroom once a day would be nice, but never really made a big deal out of not pooping as often as my boyfriend. During Burning Man 2019, I didn't poop for nine days straight. Now that I know what I know (that all the toxins trying to leave my body got reabsorbed by sitting in my gut for over a week), I definitely care more about how often I poop.

Although everyone is different, not going to the bathroom regularly could be a sign of small intestinal bacterial overgrowth (SIBO), intestinal methanogen overgrowth (IMO), inflammatory bowel disease (IBD), irritable bowel syndrome (IBS), hormone imbalances, or a bad diet.

I have noticed that, for women, our bowel habits are often linked to our sense of safety. When I went through a breakup with my partner of four years (spoiler alert: we both got emotionally healthier and got back together, so this story has a happy ending) and I was staying at an Airbnb between homes, my sense of perceived safety crumbled, and I couldn't get myself to go to the bathroom. It was as if my body was trying to hold on to *literally everything* to maintain a semblance of control.

During that time, I sat with ayahuasca, the indigenous plant medicine; she said so clearly to me: "You need to let that shit go. It's time." What came to me was a vision of me holding on to the past, to the idea of what Jacob and I used to be, who I used to be. I was desperately trying to cling to all of that.

Ever since that ayahuasca experience, I can hear her voice saying, "Let that shit go" every time I know I have to surrender. Not surprisingly, I have never had an issue going to the bathroom since then. My body and mind work together to release whatever needs to exit my life—sometimes literally.

One of the supplements we sell at Biohacking Bestie is a blend of soluble and insoluble fiber, which we call "Time to Give a Sh*t" to help you do exactly that.

(I want to add here that another way of cleansing your system is a digital detox, where you allow your mind and body to detox from the constant stream of information and screen exposure. Embracing detoxification as a lifestyle rather than a temporary fix is the ultimate biohack in managing your hormones.)

Y: Yet

You may not be ready to introduce a lot of these biohacks ... yet! That's okay! Remember, we are not aiming for perfection, only for 1% better than before. Out of the CLEAN BODY detoxifying framework, pick one to commit to as a starting point. This is about YOU, not anyone else.

For example, I had my breasts done over ten years ago. When people ask me if I'm planning on explanting them because "Now that you're a biohacker, you have to," I don't say "No"—I say "Not yet." I check myself (especially my heavy metal levels) regularly, and so far, nothing is alarming, so going through surgery and taking antibiotics feels more invasive to me at this point. I'm definitely open to it in the future. Just not yet.

Biohacking is a process that is not black and white. Remember what I said way up at the very beginning of this book: "Don't let anyone shame you for 'still' doing something." You are a person who makes her own choices and rules her own life; remember that, and make the choices that resonate most with you right now, and reserve the right to exercise the power of "yet" when you feel the need.

Avoid Toxic People

You may think it's funny that I mention toxic people in the toxins chapter, but *dang!* Don't they just drain your energy, create unnecessary drama, and engage in manipulative or abusive tactics that honestly make you feel as equally depleted as having heavy metals in your body? Cleaning up your diet *and* your circle are equally important.

Removing toxic people from your life can be challenging, but it is an essential step toward creating a healthier and more positive environment for yourself.

It's important to identify toxic behaviors and patterns. This can include constant negativity, manipulation, disrespect, gaslighting, and other consistently draining behaviors that drain your emotional or physical energy.

If you grew up in a home where this behavior was normal, you may think toxic people are the norm. They are not. I'm sorry if this is what you were taught by example. Relationships should feel supportive and expansive, and you should feel celebrated.

Establish clear boundaries and let the toxic person know what behaviors are unacceptable and what consequences will follow if they continue these behaviors. Be firm and consistent in enforcing boundaries.

Limit your interactions with toxic people as much as possible. This might involve minimizing communication, avoiding certain events or gatherings where they are present, or even cutting off contact completely if the toxicity is severe.

Talk to trusted friends, family members, or a therapist about your experiences. They can provide emotional support, guidance, and an objective perspective. Please, please, please prioritize your well-being and invest time and energy in activities that bring you joy, peace, and fulfillment. Engage in self-care practices like exercise, mindfulness, hobbies, and spending time with positive and supportive people.

Surround yourself with people who uplift and inspire you. Seek out healthy relationships that support your personal growth and well-being. In some cases, removing toxic people from your life may require ending the relationship entirely. This can be challenging, especially if the person is a family member or long-time friend.

However, prioritizing your mental and emotional well-being is crucial. Remember, removing toxic people from your life is an act of self-love and self-preservation. Initially, it may be difficult, but ultimately, it will create space for healthier relationships and a more positive and fulfilling life. I promise.

KEY TAKEAWAYS

- Avoid inflammatory foods and toxins: Steer clear of obesogens, seed oils, and glyphosate in processed foods, certain plastics, and pesticides.

- Limit exposure to heavy metals and anti-nutrients: Choose fish low in mercury, prefer organic produce, and prepare foods to reduce anti-nutrient effects.

- Follow the C-L-E-A-N B-O-D-Y Detoxification Framework: Embrace cleaner lifestyle choices; support liver and gut health; exercise regularly; and integrate adaptogens, supplements, and fasting.

- Recognize the emotional/physical health link: Emotional states significantly affect bodily functions, particularly digestion and bowel habits.

- Distance yourself from toxic people: Establish boundaries and surround yourself with supportive relationships for mental and emotional health.

- Gradually implement biohacking practices: Approach biohacking at your pace, focusing on gradual improvement and openness to future changes.

LEVEL 3:
EMBRACE YOUR CYCLE

CHAPTER 6

THE FORCE IS WITH YOU

Wow, look at you go! You've made it through Levels 1 and 2, so you now know when to eat and what your best choices are for those times when you're *not* bio-slacking. Now, you made it to Level 3. This one is probably my favorite, so buckle up! Actually, on second thought, don't buckle up—get ready to soar, because this is the level where you are about to unleash some pretty spectacular powers you may not have even realized you had.

Almost every superhero movie has the same script: someone has a special ability that they think is their curse because it makes them different from the rest of the world. They hate it until they meet someone who helps them understand that the gift is not a curse; it's a superpower.

In fact, this storyline extends even beyond the superhero genre. Take Luke Skywalker from *Star Wars*. Initially, Luke has little understanding of the Force (his gift). Only once he begins training with his mentors, Obi-Wan Kenobi and Yoda, does he become a powerful Jedi who is, ultimately, unstoppable. Or think about Elsa from *Frozen*. Initially, Elsa sees her ice powers as a curse and tries to suppress them. Once she learns to embrace them, however, she becomes incredibly powerful.

Well, guess what? You are the superhero. And what you think is your kryptonite—your cycle, your hormones, and this annoying thing that happens once a month that you are often embarrassed about (your period)—is your gift and your superpower. Let's just say the Dark Force brainwashed you to think otherwise, so you don't step into your full power.

But time for a plot twist. (Dun-dun-*DUUUUN!*)

Let finding this book be your version of meeting Obi-Wan Kenobi and the beginning of your superhero journey. You're here to leave the legacy of love, nurture, and softness only women can birth into this world, so buckle up and prepare to meet your "weapons": your hormones. Let's teach you how to use them for good.

Endocrine System

First, you need to meet the endocrine system. The endocrine system is a girl band of glands and organs that, as women's hormone expert and book author Dr. Alissa Vitti brilliantly put it, "Communicate with each other via the chemical language called hormones." However, they often metabolize (aka our body gets rid of them) through the liver, gut, and skin.

There are over 50 types of hormones in your body. Some of the most important ones, which I am sure you have heard of, are:

- Insulin (the sugar hormone)
- Oxytocin (the love and cuddles hormone)
- Serotonin (the happy, feel-good hormone)
- Dopamine (the hormone of give me more!)
- Adrenaline (the excitement hormone)

- Cortisol (the stress hormone)
- Estrogen (the feminizing/wellness hormone)
- Testosterone (the male hormone)
- Progesterone (the calming/pregnancy hormone)
- Melatonin (the sleep hormone)

When we get acne or notice weight gain or suffer painful periods, we often assume that only our sex hormones are struggling, but the truth is they are so interconnected that you will likely struggle to feel good, manage stress, or sleep right at the same time.

We live in a world full of endocrine disruptors (a fancy way of saying "a pile of absolute toxins") that confuse our body's hormonal system and get everything out of whack.

When we say, "My hormones are off," we are really saying, "My glands and organs are having communication issues." When the other chemicals mess up the communication among our organs, we call them endocrine disruptors.

Hormone/Endocrine Disruptors

There are many products, toxins, and foods in your environment that can disrupt your menstrual cycle. A few of the really big ones include:

- Consuming nonorganic produce
- Eating meat that isn't antibiotic-free and hormone-free
- Eating farmed fish
- Touching store receipts, or even worse, touching store receipts after using hand sanitizer as your skin absorbs even more BPAs
- Drinking from plastic bottles: (apparently the average person living in the Western world can consume up to a credit card-sized amount of plastic every week)

- Using chemical-laden household cleaning products and detergents
- Using drugstore cosmetics and skin care products
- Using standard nail polish and air care products that aren't all-natural
- Using tampons and pads that aren't organic
- Wearing fake fragrances rather than utilizing natural scents
- Drinking tap water

Yeah. I know it's *a lot*. Don't freak out. There are ways around all this, and that's why we are here.

First, let's see how to recognize that your hormones are off.

Some signs of a hormonal imbalance and not living according to your cycle include:

- Mood swings
- Weight gain—particularly around the hips or belly area
- PMSing
- Painful periods (which can be a sign of endometriosis, PCOS, etc.)
- Sore breasts
- Bloating
- Poor sleep quality
- Fatigue
- Cravings
- Abnormal hair growth
- Irregular cycles
- Acne
- Lack of motivation and energy

The tricky part is that these symptoms can also be due to toxins in the environment, but let's focus on hormones for right now.

Hormone Hierarchy

All hormones are *not* created equal. In her book *The Hormone Fix*, Anna Cabeca explains the hormone hierarchy and how some of them almost "override" others.

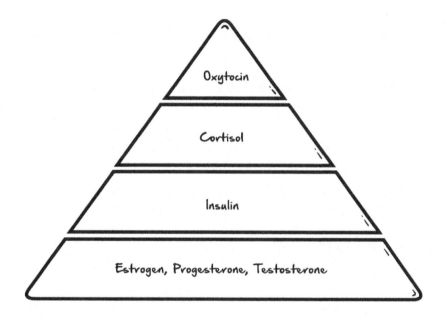

Oxytocin—the "Love Hormone"

Oxytocin is sometimes called the queen of hormones, and it's definitely one that is easy to feel and boost—plus it feels so damn good! Often dubbed the "love hormone" because it gets boosted (together with serotonin) when hugging, snuggling, petting your dog, or having sex, it does more than just make you feel warm and fuzzy. It acts like a master tuner for your body and mind, setting the stage for better hormone regulation. Boosting your oxytocin levels is more than just a feel-good hack; it's a biohack that helps maintain a balanced endocrine system. Don't worry, we'll dive into some fun and impactful ways to amp up your oxytocin levels later on!

Cortisol—the Stress Hormone

Cortisol often gets labeled as a bad guy, but I prefer to think of it as that friend who is amazing in small doses but is a bit much when they overstay their welcome. (Yeah, you know which one I'm talking about.) When life throws a curveball at you, whether from a last-minute project or when you almost have an accident, cortisol kicks in like, "Hold my purse, I've got this!" That's great, right? Of course, it is. Cortisol's got your back!

The issue arises when cortisol decides to stick around for the after-party and the after-after-party … and then just seems to be camping out on your sofa indefinitely. When those cortisol levels stay high because we're constantly in "go mode," it messes with everything from your mood and energy to your weight. Let's be real, mama: we are no strangers to stress, but knowing how to manage cortisol (and setting up boundaries with that one friend) is a total game changer.

Insulin—the Sugar Hormone

We dove into glucose in the other chapter, but I want you to understand the difference between insulin and glucose. Glucose is a type of sugar you get from the foods you eat, and it's your body's primary energy source. Think of it like the fuel for your car—without it, you're not going anywhere.

Insulin, on the other hand, is the hormone produced by your pancreas that acts like a gatekeeper. Its job is to help your cells absorb glucose from the bloodstream. Imagine it as a key that unlocks your car's fuel tank; without the key (insulin), the fuel (glucose) can't get in, and the car won't run properly. Glucose is what you need to function, and insulin allows your body to use it effectively, which is why it is so important that your insulin levels are healthy.

The Sex Hormones

Our sex hormones are like siblings. Wait—that sounds really awkward. I just mean that the hormones that can impact our bodies in ways connected to male- or femaleness are similar and live symbiotically together, but they are separate personalities that like different things.

For example, my sister is a brunette who loves baking, watching action movies, and spending time at home.

I am the exact opposite. I am a blonde who never bakes and doesn't like watching movies, but am a social butterfly who loves skydiving and spends 300 days *away* from home.

If my sister and I go to a restaurant, I'm going to order a steak, salad, and coffee. My sister will have pasta, dessert, and chamomile tea.

We love very different things. But we are still sisters (*Right, Mom? This isn't going to be the thing that sparks some big confession, is it?*), and certain things would make us both happy.

Imagine Estrogen and Progesterone Are Sisters

Estrogen is a lot like me: a go-getter, super active, adventurous, outgoing, loves-pushing-herself type who can absolutely scarf down a good steak.

Progesterone is a lot like my sister: more of a homebody who loves spending time by herself in the kitchen, nurturing herself and those around her, prioritizing restful time alone, and loves the hell out of some carbs. (Hello, premenstrual cravings!)

They also have a brother, testosterone, who shows up around ovulation to make sure we procreate and extend the species. Testosterone can be a little wild sometimes, but he's still an important group member.

Estrogen

Estrogen (who is a lot like me) is enamored with all things "fun and exciting," and she loves pushing you out of your comfort zone.

She is the bestie of womanhood, making you taller, giving you beautiful curves, and preparing your body for all the exciting adventures that lie ahead.

Progesterone

Progesterone (who is a lot like my sister) adores all things "calm and cozy," and she loves to create a peaceful atmosphere for your body to feel at ease. As a nurturer, she prepares your uterus for a potential baby guest. She's also there to make you feel calm and collected.

Testosterone

While testosterone is primarily a male hormone, it also plays essential roles in the female body. Women have much lower levels of testosterone compared to men, but they still need it to serve various functions that contribute to overall health and well-being.

Testosterone peaks around ovulation (that's why we are so horny), supports our ovaries, and boosts metabolism. Imbalances or excessive levels of testosterone, however, can lead to health issues. For example, conditions like polycystic ovary syndrome (PCOS) can be associated with higher-than-normal testosterone levels, leading to symptoms such as irregular periods, acne, and excess facial hair. All too often, women are prescribed the pill for symptoms like these that may be the result of endocrine disruptors rather than just a flare-up.

The Pill (Content Warning: Suicidal Ideation)

The birth control pill has simultaneously liberated and sickened women all over the world. It is an amazing invention with a complicated relationship to women's health.

Have you ever wondered about the real cost of that tiny pill you swallow daily? It has unquestionably changed the lives of countless women. But here's a shocker—FDA approved it for use for a few years in a woman's life, not the extended decades many of us have been taking it.

When I asked for the pill, my doctor didn't think twice. She also didn't warn me about the possible side effects. And—*wow*—there are many.

My decision about the pill was not an informed one at all. I went to the doctor because I was desperate not to get pregnant, plus I thought my period was gross and wildly inconvenient. It was also never celebrated by my then-partner: "Oh, you're on your period again? Ewww." I was not in tune with my body's intelligence, wasn't my womb's best ally, and didn't have the courage to stand up for myself. I was putting my trust in doctors, the medical system, the government, and the pharmaceutical companies, assuming they would never release a drug that would be bad for me. Boy, I was wrong.

At first, I loved not having my period, which (at that time) was more like a pain in the butt than something I celebrated. But over the next few months, I grew more and more depressed until I genuinely questioned whether I wanted to live. "I wouldn't mind dying right now," I said more than once. "Actually, I think it's a great idea."

I had broken up with my old, period-shaming, man-child of a partner and started dating my eventual-fiancé, and this side of me terrified him. "You can't be serious. Please don't ever say these words ever again," Jacob pleaded with me, not sure if I was being serious. But I was. I couldn't think of a good enough reason to stick around. It took me another month of this zombie-like state of depression until I decided to stop taking the pill. Sure enough, my suicidal thoughts stopped not long later. I am not alone. One study found that the most commonly reported reason for women to go off the pill was depression.

I'm not here to convince you to get off the pill or shame you for using it. I'm here to share with you a few facts your doctor should have communicated to you before prescribing it.

Birth control pills work their "magic" by flooding your system with synthetic hormones, tricking your body into thinking it's constantly in a pre-pregnancy state. The result? You're robbing yourself of one of nature's most powerful events: ovulation.

When you are on the pill, you're not ovulating. And I bet no one told you ovulation is your secret weapon. It's not just about potential motherhood; it's your body's periodic rev-up, making you sharper, more energetic, more *you*. However, the narrative that ties menstruation only to womanhood and motherhood is outdated and reductive.

Ovulation is your unfair advantage over men. It gives you an extra boost that makes you magnetic, healthier, and stronger. Telling a woman she doesn't need to ovulate unless she wants kids is like telling a guy he doesn't need to ejaculate unless he's ready to become a father. (From a biohacking perspective, it would actually be healthier for men to ejaculate less and for women to ovulate more, but that's a story for another book.) Long story short, we need ovulation.

On top of that, when you are on the pill, you are not producing progesterone—the "feel good" hormone. You know those times when you're totally in sync with yourself, feeling calm and centered even when the world's gone mad? Thank progesterone. This incredible hormone is produced after ovulation and has a magical way of mingling with your brain's gamma-aminobutyric acid (GABA) receptor. GABA's whole vibe is about calmness and relaxation. If you're into enneagram types, GABA is a 9 who wants to curl up with a weighted blanket and a naturally scented beeswax candle or some incense sticks. Progesterone basically says, "Yes, and let me bring you some chamomile tea and get you a deep tissue massage while we're at it." Progesterone acts as nature's very own de-stress button.

While progesterone is created naturally in your body, progestin (so close, and yet, so far) is cooked up in labs and is the main ingredient in many birth control methods. One of the most used progestins? Levonorgestrel. Structurally, it's more like testosterone than our own progesterone, and this can sometimes result in side effects that are more "male hormone" than "female hormone" — think potential hair loss or weight gain. Your body is designed for one, but ends up getting an almost-but-not-really substitute. It's like expecting a quiet coffee date and getting a rock concert instead.

Not everyone experiences these challenging physical responses, but it's important to be aware that these man-made hormones can screw up your natural hormones, even (especially) insulin. Ironically, while natural estrogen in your body helps your insulin response, the pill's synthetic counterpart makes you more likely to have a glucose spike. That's right — the pill can also mess with how your body handles sugar! Some studies suggest that the synthetic hormones in it (like estrogen and insulin) can interact in ways that cause insulin resistance in women. This means that your body might struggle to use insulin correctly, which can cause high blood sugar levels.

The pill also sucks life-essential minerals like folic acid, selenium, and zinc from your system. The ripple effect? Hormonal chaos, troubled skin, bloating, and sneaky weight gain.

Again, I am not here to shame you about your choices. I just want to raise some questions and your awareness about some serious issues you may not have been properly warned about. For example, did your doctor tell you that the pill can influence your ability to respond to men's pheromones, and you might end up choosing the wrong partner?

When Hollywood director Abby Epstein and legendary talk show host Ricki Lake came on my podcast to talk about their movie *The Business of Birth Control*, Abby shared that after she stopped taking the pill, she felt "repulsed" by her partner. "And I'm not the only one, Aggie," she went on. "Many, many women we interviewed stopped being attracted to their partner after they got off the pill, which is usually when they try for a baby."

After several years of being off the pill, I am happy to report that I am in a healthy and passionate relationship with a man I find deeply attractive and who celebrates my period even more than I do. He doesn't shy away from it but, rather, treats it like a guest of honor at our play dates. Men who act like periods are unnatural and gross either need to grow up, man up, or educate themselves. Your period is a miracle and should be celebrated and welcomed as such.

If there is one takeaway you keep from this book, let it be this: You are your own Prince(ss) Charming. You need to look out for, question, double check, and critique everything you hear and check with your internal compass—including the preferences I shared with you here. Protect *yourself*. Question. Observe. Test things. See for yourself.

The notion that menstruation defines womanhood or motherhood is outdated and unfair. If you are reading this and you haven't had your period for a while, I want to remind you that your worth as a woman extends far beyond your reproductive capabilities. We need to write a new narrative about what defines being a woman that goes way beyond simply being a mom, and having ovaries or breasts.

Being a woman is an energy—a frequency you can tap into. And whether you are on the pill, have a period, or not, I highly encourage you to live according to your own cycle—whatever that looks like.

Your Infradian Rhythm

I often see fitness experts who share how much they love their exercise and diet plan, only to share in passing that they haven't had their period in years! Your period is one of the most important guides of your hormonal cycles and is considered your fifth vital sign, alongside body temperature, pulse rate, respiration rate, and blood pressure. This means menstruation is one of the body's main ways of indicating what your hormonal balance is doing. If your period is irregular, skipped, delayed, extremely heavy, painful, or stops altogether without a clear explanation, it's time to take it very seriously. No matter what kind of "Suck it up, buttercup" advice you've been given in the past about your period, you need to know that painful periods are *not normal*.

Your Cycle: What Is Normal, Anyway?

Everyone's cycle is unique to them, but it's important to be sure that yours is in the realm of "normal." The length of your cycle should last somewhere between 28 to 32 days—anywhere in between is fine as long as it is regular and consistent for you. Ideally, your period should last four to seven days.

So how do you track your hormone levels to know where you stand, especially if you are sensing signs and symptoms that something might be off—and what can help you get them back into balance? When I was doing research on hormones, I found that so much of the data out there is geared toward menopausal women, which is great for them, but not very helpful for those of us who aren't at that stage of life yet.

Infra ... What?

I was 34 when I first heard the term "infradian" rhythm. As a bio-hacker, I knew about circadian rhythm (our daily 24-hour rhythm), but infradian rhythm was very new.

Different from the circadian rhythm, the infradian rhythm is your monthly rhythm. It is your internal, 28-day cycle that regulates the menstrual cycle, which ancient cultures realized mirrored the moon. As women, our superpower is the fact we are synced up with nature. We can try to fight it and feel terrible or dance along with it and feel like goddesses.

We are obviously not men, yet our society is built around a man's cycle, which is rooted in the circadian rhythm (aka a daily cycle). Men's hormones are much like the sun; testosterone goes up in the morning and drops in the afternoon.

By contrast, women are lunar. It's no coincidence that the length of our menstrual cycles is synced up with the waxing and waning of the moon, occurring around every 28 days. Our rhythm, rather than being exclusively circadian, is both circadian *and* infradian. (Look at our amazing bodies naturally multitasking like boss ass bitches!)

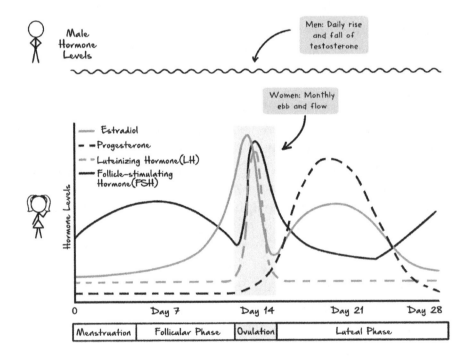

As you can clearly see, our hormones are not anywhere near the same as men's. In fact, they are almost never the same for even a few consecutive days.

We are like rivers: constantly flowing and changing. If you aren't supporting your cycle, you are most likely working against it.

Energy Cycling (Yin and Yang)

One of the many reasons I love living according to my cycle is that I can cycle between the yin and yang energies throughout the month instead of trying to fit them all into one day. Actually, it's how our bodies have been designed.

Yin and yang? I am sure you have heard about them before. Chinese philosophy delves into the idea that opposite forces aren't just interconnected but are also complementary. One can't live without the other.

Masculine energy (yang) is often about doing. It's that force that drives you to achieve, solve problems, and take action. It's interested in the "how" and "why" of things. Yang energy loves a good challenge and is often focused on winning or improving. Think of discipline, rules, and frameworks. Yang energy loves a well-organized plan.

Feminine energy (yin), on the other hand, is more about being. It's open, willing to receive, and focused on the present moment. This is the energy that guides you when you "just know" something but can't explain why. Yin is intuition and deep inner wisdom. Unlike competitive yang energy, yin is all about cooperation and community. It's more fluid and adaptable. It's like water; it can adjust to the shape of any container it finds itself in.

There is a big misconception that women should only live in feminine energy and men should stick to being strictly masculine.

That comes from the notion of "You're my other half; you complete me." If, as a woman, I can only tap into the feminine energy, I have to rely on my partner to get things done for me, to bring stability, and to offer direction; this means I can't experience true agenda-less love, because I need my partner to survive. There is an expectation to fulfill—a condition that has to be met. A woman who can't tap into the healthy masculine energy in her life sets herself up for codependency and denies herself the gift of being a whole person.

We are here to be whole. Everyone has both yin and yang energies, regardless of gender. The trick is finding the balance. Too much yang and you might find yourself stressed, overly competitive, and burnt out. Too much yin and you might end up feeling unproductive or stuck in a rut.

So, for example, if you're grinding 24/7 (yang to the max), you might need to tap into some yin by doing some deep breathing, meditating, or even just taking a chill day. Conversely, if you're feeling lethargic or unmotivated (too much yin), it might be time to activate that yang energy with some goal-setting or a kick-butt workout.

We want to experience both masculine and feminine energies within each one of us so we don't need our partner to survive. Instead, we want to choose our partner to stand next to us to love us unconditionally—and vice versa.

Meet Your Cycle

As women, we have four phases in the 28-day cycle.

Phase 1: Menstrual Phase/Inner Winter: Yin energy, inward focus, reflection, intuition, active rest

Phase 2: Follicular Phase/Inner Spring: Yang energy, outward focus, curiosity, taking action, loving discipline and structure, competition with yourself

Phase 3: Ovulatory Phase/Inner Summer: Peak of yang energy, achievement, attraction, drive (including sexual), peak energy, chasing after your dreams

Phase 4: Luteal Phase/Inner Fall: Yin energy, inward focus, self-reflection, tuning into emotional needs, heightened intuition, attracting instead of chasing

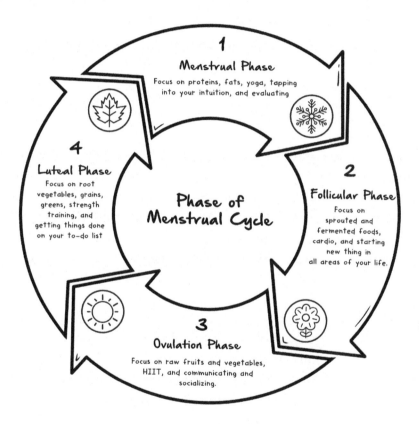

Sync With the Moon

If you are a woman who is postmenopausal, doesn't have a period, or is on the pill, you can still sync up with the moon's cycle and start the Phase 1 steps on the first day of the new moon. These practices still align with your natural rhythms and can serve as a beautiful celebration of your female-ness as you follow the ancient wisdom of honoring the moon's natural waning and waxing.

Phase 1: Menstrual Phase/Inner Winter

Yin energy, inward focus, reflection, intuition, active rest.

- Time to shed anything that isn't serving you.
- Reconnect with the wild woman within.
- Time to remember you already possess all answers inside yourself.

Timing

Days 1-7

Phase 1 is the day when your period starts up to about Day 7 (this might vary by a day or two). This is the time of your cycle for you to remember who the f*ck you are and connect with your nature. Your raw medicine woman is untamed but grounded. She is part of the cycle of life as the life-giver. Every time you have your period, remember your true power and the beautiful gift that you have been given.

Biology

When our estrogen and progesterone drop, they signal to your body that it's time to start shedding the uterine lining. The uterine lining that was built up in preparation for a potential pregnancy now exits the body through the vagina. This is, you know, the actual "period" part. You might experience cramps due to uterine contractions, fatigue because of hormone shifts, and other symptoms like headaches or tender breasts.

Energy

In line with the yin energy, you might feel a natural inclination to slow down, reflect, and take it easy. Since you are already shedding, this is also time to release situations, people, and dynamics that aren't serving your Higher Self.

If you follow me on Instagram, you may notice I usually don't post for two or three days each month. *Now you know why!* I try to take this time to regroup and ask myself what really matters and what is actually important to me right now. This is the time to fill my own cup, instead of filling others—a time to look within and reconnect with my Higher Self.

I want to encourage you to get comfortable with the discomfort of this time. It's okay if you take a painkiller every now and then, but try not to make it a habit. As Brené Brown says, "We cannot selectively numb emotions." If you numb sadness, you will also numb joy. If you numb pain, you will numb pleasure and ecstasy. We get touchy, and maybe we don't like feeling anything that isn't fun, but our true growth is in our shadow—the part of us that is hard to love and accept. This is a beautiful monthly challenge nature extends to us; I love going inward and trying to love myself when I am not being super productive. I'd love for you to embrace this opportunity, as well. And if the pain is really unbearable—this is a sign to see your doctor ASAP.

Diet

This phase of your cycle loves a clean keto diet without dairy: focus on fats and protein. Think grass-fed steak and organ meats to make stews, and enjoy good fats like avocados, butter, coconut, and olive oil. Also, be sure to include hearty leafy greens, vegetables, dark-colored berries, and trace minerals. Limit your carbs and try to avoid all sugar.

Fasting

As your estrogen levels start to rise, they can potentially make fasting feel more manageable. Start with shorter fasts and gradually increase the fasting window as you get further away from the day of your period, being mindful of your body and waiting until the immediate effects of your period subside. Start with a shorter fast, perhaps in the 13-16 hour range, and then gradually extend it up to as long as 72 hours if you're experienced with fasting and feel good doing so.

Exercise

This is not the time to push yourself and aim for your personal best, but it's not the time to glue yourself to the couch, either.

Low-impact cardio: Think walking, cycling, or swimming. These low-impact exercises can boost your mood and endurance without being too taxing on the body.

Yoga and stretching: Some gentle yoga poses can help with cramps and bloating. Just maybe avoid the inversions; they can sometimes feel uncomfortable when you're on your period.

Bodyweight exercises: Think squats, lunges, or push-ups. If you're not feeling super energetic, bodyweight exercises can be a great way to stay active without overexerting yourself.

Pilates: This is another low-impact option that focuses on core strength and flexibility, which can be especially good if you're experiencing back pain along with menstrual cramps.

Light weightlifting: If you're up for it, some light-to-moderate weightlifting can also be beneficial. Just avoid going for your max reps during this time.

Lifestyle

Give yourself permission to let your womb decide what feels right. If staying home and snuggling up on the couch is what you need, honor that. You can use this time to catch up on meditation and journaling as well as practice manifesting to attract anything you want, remembering that in the quantum field, it's already yours and was always meant to be.

Sex

Menstruation doesn't mean you shouldn't have sex, but some women are not really into it at this point in their cycle. I mentioned that energetically we go within, which means that we tend to crave *intimacy* more than we crave sex right now. The true connection with our partner is what really turns us on and makes us feel seen, as opposed to a quickie or maintenance sex.

In my app, Cycle Bestie, we share some ideas to connect with your partner on a deeper level without penetration and suggest some fun, sexy positions you can try out!

Side note: The way to tell a boy from a man is this: boys are afraid of or grossed out by periods, make fun of them, and want nothing to do with them. Men cherish, celebrate, and love their woman's period. Plus, you are not fertile when you're on your period, so if you are trying to avoid pregnancy, you can really go for it if you want! And if you don't want to, that's okay, too! A lot of women prefer self-pleasure around this time. *But what about the mess?* Girl, darker sheets, towels, and that amazing little invention called a washing machine has been my go-to. So you have a little extra laundry to do—what's that compared to a chance to let your body seek pleasure however she wants it rather than feeling ashamed of something perfectly natural?

Cervical Fluid

You know those fortune tellers who do readings from tea leaves? Well, that can be you, except you'll be reading your health from the color of your period blood. Look at you being all magical!

Remember that the color of your period can be affected by many factors, including diet, exercise, age, contraceptive use, and overall health. During your period itself, you may notice several different types of flow:

Bright red or crimson—indicates a normal, healthy flow. Congrats! You've got a happy vag.

Dark red or burgundy—usually occurs at the beginning or end of the menstrual cycle. It's older blood that takes longer to leave the uterus and is nothing to worry about. Again, well done on the hearty lady bits.

Brown or black—usually seen at the end of the period when the blood is older and has had time to oxidize. It's often seen in the morning after lying down all night. This can sometimes happen with spotting at the very beginning of your cycle as well, as your body clears out any blood that didn't quite clear the system last time. It's usually not a cause for concern.

Pink—may mean low estrogen levels, poor nutrition, or intense exercise. It could also be a sign of anemia. Think about what changes you can make to your activity level and nutrition to raise your iron levels or bring your hormones back in line.

Orange or dark yellow—This color could indicate an infection, especially if there is a foul smell or unusual texture. It could also be a sign of irregular menstruation, especially if it occurs along with other symptoms like pain, burning, itching, or unusual discharge. Keep an eye on things and contact a healthcare provider if something doesn't feel right.

Gray—Gray discharge could be a sign of bacterial vaginosis or other infections. If you're seeing gray, especially if it's accompanied by a foul smell or fever, you should contact a healthcare provider immediately. Please prioritize your health.

Keep in mind that your cervical mucus changes throughout your cycle. Right after your period ends, your cervical mucus or vaginal discharge will be white or yellow-tinged and will feel dry or tacky.

Biohacks for a Better Period

- Castor oil packs or heating pads (These provide a gentle way of improving blood flow to the organs in your pelvis, but don't use them if you have a heavy flow.)
- Journaling
- Meditation
- Lymphatic drainage
- Dry brushing

Mantra for Phase 1

"I am not missing out on anything. I don't have FOMO (fear of missing out); I have JOMO (joy of missing out)."

Phase 2: Follicular Phase/Inner Spring

Yang energy, outward focus, curiosity, taking action

- Remind the world about your legacy
- Loving discipline and structure
- You will become a little competitive, but remember the only competition is always between you and you.

Timing

Days 7-11 of your cycle

Biology

Your estrogen is on the rise, prepping your uterus for a possible pregnancy, while the follicle-stimulating hormone (FSH) gets to work in your ovaries to mature a new batch of eggs. Estrogen has a stimulating effect, so you're likely to feel a boost in energy. It's like your body's natural espresso shot. Many women find they're sharper and more focused during this phase. Physically, you may notice a progressive strengthening in your stamina and muscle tone.

Energy

As you step into your inner spring phase, it's like someone just hit the "refresh" button on your energy. You'll feel lighter and more adventurous, and there's an undeniable magnetic pull toward socializing and connection. It's spring after all! It's a time to birth new ideas, expand your horizons, and follow your curiosity down whatever rabbit hole it leads you. Embrace the playfulness that bubbles up within you—let it guide your actions and be prepared to dream big. With each passing day, you'll find yourself getting stronger, more motivated, and ready to conquer whatever comes your way. It's your time to shine, to build, and to seize the opportunities.

Diet

Estrogen improves your ability to use insulin and regulates blood sugar levels. But that doesn't mean we should abuse it! During this phase, you'll notice an increased metabolic rate. Continue with a diet focused primarily on protein and healthy fats, but given the elevated energy and focus, add a broader spectrum of fresh vegetables into your meals. We're going for slightly lighter foods that are easy to digest yet packed with nutrients—think protein bowls, salads, berries, cacao, and plenty of good protein (organ meat, steak, lamb, and fish). Opt for nutrient-dense veggies such as zucchini, broccoli, and Brussels sprouts, along with a splash of color from carrots. Fruits like berries and citrus fruits (particularly lemon, lime, and grapefruit) can complement your diet with natural sweetness and vital antioxidants. For nuts and seeds, focus on pumpkin, flax, Brazil nuts, and cashews to add both texture and essential fatty acids to your meals. A range of herbs such as parsley, nettle, and holy basil can add not only flavor but also potential health benefits. Fermented foods like pickled veggies, sauerkraut, and kimchi also add flavor as well as support gut health.

Advanced biohackers aim for this macro breakdown: 15% carbs, 25% protein, 60% fats.

Fasting

Ever wanted to push yourself when fasting? Well, the time is now. If you are new to fasting, start by extending your fast by one to two hours on Day 7 and then pushing it an extra 30 minutes on the following days (or every other day if that feels like too much).

Exercise

Time to grab those heavy weights and really push yourself with high-intensity interval training (HIIT), reduced-exertion high-intensity training (REHIT), and sprint interval training (SIT). You have a higher tolerance for endurance and pain, your uptake of oxygen is increased, and you can also recover better, so you can make a lot of training progress. Time to aim for your PR (personal record) for the heaviest weights or the longest run.

Lifestyle

Leverage your heightened focus and energy levels to initiate new projects, set up client meetings, expand your network, and dive into complex tasks that require sustained attention. Use this phase as a springboard to advance your professional goals, invest in your personal growth, and make proactive lifestyle changes that align with your goals. Dream big!

Sex

Slowly but surely, you will notice yourself wanting to have sex without having to gaze for hours into your partner's eyes first. Now that we are inhabiting a more masculine energy, we may feel like "hunting" for our prey. Biologically, our brains want to keep the species going, so we may naturally feel more flirty and horny. My first advice is: flirt with life! I don't mean every guy you see. I mean *life*. Be playful, start a conversation, laugh, feel powerful, and take the opportunity life is giving you. Just remember that this is a great time to have sex, but also the trickiest. Sperm can survive up to five days in your body, and you can ovulate as early as Day 11 or 12 of your cycle, depending on how regular you are. Take the proper precautions if you are trying to avoid pregnancy.

Cervical Fluid

On Days 7-9 of your cycle, your juices will become creamy with a yogurt-like consistency. It will feel wet and cloudy down there.

Mantra for Phase 2

"My dreams were given to me for a reason. My purpose in life is to go after them."

Phase 3: Ovulatory Phase/Inner Summer

peak of yang energy, achievement, attraction, drive (also sexual), peak energy

Timing

Days 12-15 of your cycle

Biology

During ovulation, your body undergoes a series of hormonal changes that prepare it for a potential pregnancy. Your estrogen and luteinizing hormone (LH) peak around this time to facilitate the release of a mature egg from one of your ovaries into the fallopian tube. Body temperature rises slightly after the egg is released, an indicator some people use for fertility tracking. You might also find that you have heightened senses, increased energy, and even an elevated libido due to a peak in testosterone. Your pain tolerance may increase, and your overall physical performance might improve, which will make you unstoppable. (Remember when I said this was your superpower?)

Energy

During ovulation, you're in your yang energy, which is traditionally associated with attributes like action, heat, and brightness. This resonates with the physical changes and hormonal surges your body undergoes during this phase. Energetically, you may feel more outgoing, social, and motivated to tackle challenges, whether they be in your personal life, workouts, or the workplace. The increase in yang energy during ovulation can make you feel more alive, alert, and in tune with your desires and ambitions. It's a powerful time to reconnect with your personal "turn on," your sexual life-force energy. Chase hard after your dreams!

Diet

During your inner summer, when your hormones are at their peak and your body temperature is elevated, opt for raw vegetables and lighter foods to cool your body. Veggies like Brussels sprouts and broccoli are excellent choices, along with fruits such as coconut, watermelon, and berries. Proteins like wild-caught salmon and poultry can be beneficial, as well as herbs like dandelion root and turmeric. Seeds like sesame are rich in lignans and minerals that block excess estrogen, while sunflower seeds, high in selenium and vitamin E, can aid in progesterone production and support liver detoxification.

Macro breakdown: 40% carbs, 40% protein, 30% fats

Fasting

Step out of your longer fasting state and turn it down a notch. Don't fast for longer than 17 hours at a time.

Exercise

You're likely to have more energy, increased strength, and better pain tolerance during this phase. This is an ideal time for intense workouts and lifting heavier weights. Your body's increased pain tolerance can help you push through more challenging sets and make you go for your personal best. You could also opt for longer, more strenuous cardio sessions. Whether it's running, cycling, or swimming, your stamina is likely to be improved during this phase. With your social and communication skills also getting a hormonal boost, this is a great time for group exercise classes where you can feed off the energy of others.

Lifestyle

Did you know that scientists found that female strippers earn the most tips when they're ovulating? (Women on the pill earned the least.) What does it mean? During ovulation, women are considered more beautiful and more attractive. Use it to your own (un) fair advantage during this time: ask for a raise, plan your public speaking, take new headshots, or (as I plan to do) schedule your wedding!

You may also find that you're more inclined to take the lead in social situations or be more assertive in expressing your needs and desires. You feel it is easier to make decisions and take action on plans you've been contemplating. You may feel more adventurous and willing to take calculated risks, like trying out a new workout routine, tackling a new project at work, or even initiating conversations in your personal relationships that you've been putting off.

Sex

During your inner summer, reconnect with your sexual energy instead of shaming yourself for it or feeling like it's your shadow-self. It's perfectly normal to feel horny, so embrace it. It isn't wrong or bad. Tap into that energy with your want to—either with a partner or by yourself. Self-pleasure can be a big part of your empowerment. If you feel horny, enjoy it! If you are trying for a baby, this is show time. If not, make responsible decisions.

One great biohack is for your partner to learn non-ejaculatory orgasm. Yes, that is a real thing. Taoism, Ayurveda, and Tantra believe ejaculating often depletes men of their life force energy and "weakens" them, so they encourage men to learn how to climax without ejaculating. With a little bit of practice, your partner can become really good at this, which will not only improve your sex life but will also improve the way he interacts with the world.

Cervical Fluid

The mucus will be stretchy and resemble raw egg whites. The mucus gets the most slippery and stretchy just before the egg is released. You are at your most fertile, and your cervical mucus is at its peak in terms of being accommodating for sperm at this time.

Mantra for Phase 3

"I embrace my sexuality and celebrate the power of my pussy."

Phase 4: Luteal Phase/Inner Fall

Yin energy, inward focus, self-reflection, heightened intuition

Timing

1st half (Days 16-21)

2nd half (Days 22-28)

The first half of this phase (your "inner fall") is called the early luteal phase (Days 16 to 21), and the second half is the late luteal phase (Days, 21-28) which is when some women experience PMS.

Biology

During the luteal phase, which occurs after ovulation and before the start of menstruation, your estrogen first rises during the early part of the luteal phase, working in tandem with progesterone to further prepare the uterine lining. If a pregnancy does not occur, both progesterone and estrogen drop, and premenstrual symptoms like mood swings, bloating, and breast tenderness may start to present. Your basal body temperature will generally be higher.

Energy

As you transition into your yin energy during the luteal phase of your menstrual cycle, you are moving from the external to the internal. Energetically, this is when you may feel a need to slow down, conserve energy, and honor your inner emotional world. While yang energy is about building and conquering, yin energy is about nurturing and holding space for yourself. You might find it beneficial to retreat from overly social or strenuous activities and prioritize self-care and relaxation. I prefer smaller circles and deeper conversations during my luteal phase. This inward focus isn't a sign of weakness or withdrawal but, rather, a natural attunement to your body's cycles. By honoring your yin energy, you create a balance that allows for emotional and physical restoration, setting the stage for the next cycle of yang energy when the time comes.

Diet

During the first part of this phase, you can continue with low-carb intake. But as you approach the menstrual stage and your progesterone levels rise, you may find yourself craving carbohydrates more—while also becoming slightly insulin resistant. This means that a cookie that would usually cause only a small spike in your glucose now is going to have a much stronger effect on your body, which can lead to even more cravings. Chips, cookies, and pasta will only make your PMS worse; you'll end up even crampier, moodier, and hungrier. To help avoid PMS, focus on slower-burning calories, incorporating good fats and proteins, which cause less of a glucose spike.

Some experts advise not to eat any carbs because of that, but I prefer to trust the intelligence of nature. Progesterone needs good "nature" carbs, not just any carbs. Focus on carbs like pumpkin, butternut squash, squash, carrot, arrowroot, sweet potato, red potato, yam, plantain, and white rice. Veggies you might want to incorporate include cabbage, cauliflower, celery, cucumber, collard, and mustard greens. For protein, try turkey, wild-caught salmon, grass-fed beef, lamb, as well as dark chocolate. Approved sugars for the cravings include xylitol (but be careful around your pets because xylitol is lethal to dogs), erythritol, monk fruit, d-ribose, sorbitol, raw honey, and sugar alcohols like maltitol.

Advanced Biohackers:

Macro breakdown in Part 1 of this phase: 15% carbs, 25% protein, 60% fats

Macro breakdown in Part 2 of this phase: 40% carbs, 40% protein, 30% fats

Fasting

In the first part of the phase, you can still intermittently fast (I call these the "last push days"). But seven days before your period, forget about intentional fasting. Now, that doesn't mean 10 p.m. dinners (unless you're in Spain). Try to have your last meal of the day at 6-7 p.m., and then breakfast when you wake up.

Exercise

In the first half of the luteal phase, when you still have relatively more energy, a moderate approach to strength training and cardio can be great; try workouts that are neither too taxing nor too relaxed.

This allows for a harmonious transition from the high-energy follicular phase to the more introspective luteal phase.

As you get closer to menstruation, consider shifting your focus entirely toward self-care and stress relief. Pilates, yoga, and long walks become your best friends during this time. It is not a time for pushing boundaries or setting personal bests at the gym. Why? Because we want to keep cortisol—the "stress" hormone—on the lower side. Elevated cortisol levels can intensify insulin resistance, and insulin sensitivity is already naturally lowered during this phase. You can still engage in strength training but opt for lighter weights and less intense routines. Forget fasting workouts or prolonged cardio sessions; they can push your cortisol levels too high.

Lifestyle

Yang, the feminine energy, is the "receiving" one, but we modern women seem to have forgotten how to receive. We live in a world where productivity is a badge of honor. We feel broken and weak when we need to rest and recharge. Unlike the yang phase, where you might have felt more driven to initiate projects and lead teams, yin energy prompts a different kind of productivity. You may find yourself more focused on fine-tuning existing projects rather than launching new ones. It's a time for detail-oriented tasks, revising, reviewing, and reflecting. You may find yourself more in tune with the needs and feelings of your colleagues. Yin energy supports the "nurturer" role—you're great at problem-solving from a compassionate perspective, ensuring that the team's emotional and practical needs are met.

Additionally, your inclination toward self-care and stress management can be a strength in the workplace. You can set the tone for a balanced, healthy work environment by prioritizing well-being. Try suggesting shorter, more focused meetings or introducing relaxation techniques to combat workplace stress. Even though you may not be in "go-go-go" mode, your yin energy during the luteal phase can be a unique asset, helping to balance out the often yang-dominated corporate culture.

Sex

At the beginning of your luteal phase, you may be down for a quickie; but as you approach the end of the phase, you will feel more of a need for intimacy than sex. You may feel a bit dry and not super down to have sex, so try lots of coconut oil as lubrication and more time for foreplay if you do want to give it a try.

Your cervix will be lower in the second half, so if you have penetrative sex, it may be uncomfortable in certain positions (or in all of them). Remember that sex goes beyond penetration. Oral, non-penetrative sex, self-pleasure, and erotic or non-erotic massage can all meet your need for intimacy while honoring your body's comfort.

Cervical Fluid

Your cervical mucus will stay dry until menstruation occurs, so (again) make coconut oil or your lubrication of choice your best friend.

Mantra for Phase 4

"Resting is not a weakness, and receiving is not shameful."

Ways to Balance Your H-O-R-M-O-N-E-S

To make it easier to remember, use the H-O-R-M-O-N-E-S framework to think about how to support your hormones with intentionality.

H: Honor

Honor the feminine within. Support your infradian rhythm by living, eating, fasting, and working out according to your cycle. We are different from men, and it's time we embrace that. Rather than aspiring to be less hairy versions of them, let's celebrate and honor our cycles, our wombs, and our pussies. These hormones aren't just the natural chemicals your body produces; they're superpowers. Use apps (like Cycle Bestie) or journals to track your menstrual cycle, symptoms, and overall well-being. Understanding your cycle patterns can empower you to claim your power back.

O: Oxytocin

Embrace your oxytocin (love hormone) and flood yourself with these feel-good hormones that will support your entire endocrine system. It doesn't just make you feel good at the moment. By plussing up your oxytocin levels through things like snuggling, hugging, petting, kissing, and massage, you're doing more than just sparking joy. You're essentially laying the foundation for your body to find that much-needed state of equilibrium. So go ahead and go snuggle; your hormones will thank you!

R: Remove Toxins

Detox your body and support your liver. Your liver metabolizes estrogen, so it is always good to ensure you are not overloading it with other toxins, such as alcohol or processed chemicals. Try to avoid overburdening it, especially if you are already feeling that your hormones are out of balance. The same goes for your gut. Keep reading; I'll have some biohacks for you on how to detox like a pro coming up.

M: Manage Glucose

Manage glucose spikes and regulate insulin. This is one of the most efficient ways to tackle signs of a hormonal imbalance. Insulin is a hormone that will often "override" and disrupt sex hormones, but it's easy to regulate with small adjustments to your diet.

O: Optimize Your Routine

The objective is to optimize, not traumatize. The key is moderation. Biohacks like fasting and cold exposure are incredible for regulating your hormones, but their impact is highly dependent on how they're applied. Diving headlong into a 72-hour fast or spending excessive time in ice-cold water might give you bragging rights on Instagram, but it can also shock your system and throw your hormones into disarray. Start with intermittent fasting or spend just a few minutes in a cold shower before *gradually* working your way up. The goal is to gently guide your body into a state of equilibrium where hormone production is supported.

N: Nourish

Nourish is one of my favorite words on the planet. It just makes me feel so seen and safe. Women blossom when we are nourished. Make sure you are not walking around hungry; nourish your body by eating enough good fat such as avocado, seeds, ghee, coconut oil, and butter.

E: Electronics Exposure

We have become very "indoorsy" as a species, but our hormones are intricately connected to natural light. Many of us spend countless hours under the artificial glow of fluorescent lights or glued to our phone screens—from the first seconds we wake up in the morning until late at night—behaviors that are throwing our hormonal balance out of whack. It's not just melatonin, the sleep hormone, that gets affected; the damage extends through our entire endocrine system. Beyond our circadian rhythm, artificial light can mess with our infradian rhythms too! A recent study found a possible link between blue lights (such as those used in electronic screens) and premature onset of puberty.

One of the simplest biohacks is to get outside and wear blue light-blocking glasses whenever you can. Consistent exposure to natural sunlight doesn't just lift your spirits; it also helps produce vitamin D, a critical component for hormone synthesis. Considering we're probably the most sun-deprived generation in history, making a conscious effort to catch some rays isn't just a luxury—it's a necessity when managing your hormones.

S: Stress

Manage your stress. Stress is a very important factor in hormone balance, and we will deep-dive into stress in another chapter! When your cortisol is high, your sex hormones will be out of whack. If your body doesn't think it's safe out there, she won't ovulate and have a period because, once again, your biology is wired to propagate the species, and unsafe conditions aren't an ideal time to bring a new human into the world!

KEY TAKEAWAYS

- **Embrace Your Menstrual Cycle as a Superpower:** Understand and respect the different phases of your menstrual cycle—menstrual, follicular, ovulatory, and luteal—each with its unique energy and needs. This cycle is not a curse but a powerful tool for understanding your body and optimizing your health and well-being.

- **Understand the Endocrine System and Hormonal Balance:** Hormones like insulin, oxytocin, serotonin, dopamine, adrenaline, cortisol, estrogen, testosterone, progesterone, and melatonin play crucial roles in overall health. Disruptions in these hormones can manifest as mood swings, weight gain, PMS, fatigue, and more.

- **Identify and Avoid Endocrine Disruptors:** Common disruptors include nonorganic produce, hormone-laden meat and dairy, plastic containers, chemical cleaning products, and non-natural personal care items. Reducing exposure to these can significantly improve hormonal balance.

- **Honor Your Body's Natural Rhythms:** Tune into your body's infradian rhythm (your 28-day cycle) and circadian rhythm. Honor the yin and yang energies throughout the month to balance activity and rest.

- **Diet and Nutrition Adjustments According to Cycle Phases:** Adapt your diet to each phase of your cycle, focusing on different macronutrients and foods that align with your body's changing needs, from protein and fats during the menstrual phase to balanced carbs, proteins, and fats in the luteal phase.

- **Manage Stress and Emotional Well-Being:** High stress levels can disrupt hormonal balance, especially cortisol. Incorporating stress-reduction techniques like meditation, yoga, and mindful practices is crucial.

- **Regular Exercise Adapted to Menstrual Phases:** Adjust your exercise routine to match the energy levels of each menstrual phase, from low-impact activities during menstruation to more intense workouts during the follicular and ovulatory phases.

- **Technology and Light Exposure Management:** Be mindful of excessive exposure to blue light from screens, which can disrupt both circadian and infradian rhythms. Getting natural sunlight and using blue light-blocking glasses can help regulate hormones.

LEVEL 4:
LIVE LIKE A BIOHACKER

CHAPTER 7

TRAIN LIKE A BIOHACKER

"I've always believed that if you put in the work, the results will come. I don't do things half-heartedly. Because I know if I do, then I can expect half-hearted results."

—Michael Jordan

Here we are! You've made it to Level 4! You now know when to time your meals, what your most nutritious choices are, and how to work with your cycle to celebrate your female superpower! Let's take a look at how it all comes together with some final bio-hacking touches as you embrace your new identity and transform into your most powerful self! Let's start with training.

Strong > Skinny

Now, it's the fun part. You have been eating like a biohacker, looking at your hormones as a biohacker, and now it's time to live like one. As biohackers, we love moving our bodies, but we don't live at the gym. We do workouts that actually move the needle, not just spend hours in classes for the sake of saying we spent time at the gym.

My goal used to be to see how skinny I could get. I thought that was all that mattered. When I got my weight down to 40 kgs (about 89 pounds; I'm only 5' 3, but still), I thought I would be on top of the world, full of energy, and everything would be great. But I found that I wasn't feeling strong, and I wasn't toned. Since I didn't want to get bulky like a gym bro, I was afraid of lifting weights.

My mindset of "the skinnier, the better" makes me cringe now. I don't weigh myself very often anymore; in fact, I don't even own a scale. I know that as a woman, my weight fluctuates according to my period, what I eat, and water retention—there are a dozen different reasons. I don't want to spend my life obsessing over a natural fluctuation of a pound or two. I don't like the term "losing weight," even though I do use it in this book because it is commonly used to mean "getting fit," but I really want you to understand that *these are often not the same thing*.

In biohacking, we measure body composition and prioritize muscle because they make being fit so much easier.

When I was at my "skinniest," I was not fit. I had very little muscle. You can be any weight and be fit if you are packing a healthy amount of *muscle* and your body systems are working as they should. In my signature biohacking challenge, Fit as F*ck, where I have coached over 20,000 women (and counting), a lot of women come with the goal of losing weight, but they quickly understand how much easier that's going to be when they build muscle first.

Not everyone wants or likes the athletic look of a bubble butt, but that's not what we are talking about here. I want you to focus on strong skeletal muscles, which are necessary to thrive physically.

First of all, fat is less metabolically active than muscle. This means a kilogram of fat burns fewer calories at rest than a kilogram of muscle. Muscle tissue is metabolically active, which means it requires more energy (calories) to maintain itself, even when you're at rest. On top of that, remember: the more muscle, the more insulin receptors you have to store insulin during a carby meal, which means fewer glucose spikes. The fewer glucose spikes, the better you feel. The better you feel, the more energy you have to do the things you love. See where I'm going with this?

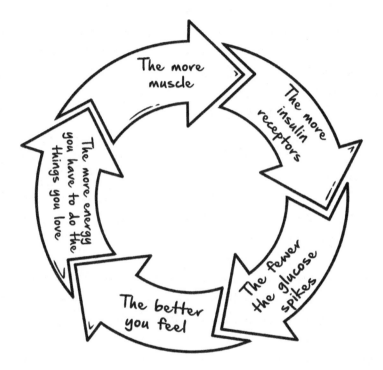

Remember, *we are not here to lose weight*. Well, let me rephrase that slightly: we are *not* here to gauge our worth by a number on the scale. We *are* here to lose the weight we put on ourselves with endless responsibilities where we might feel like we are always failing to measure up: house, job, kids, thinking we are responsible for everyone else's happiness and well-being. *That* is the weight that manifests in our fat cells (more on that later). It's time to look at the weight of these external pressures and drop it like it's hot. (Thanks for that sage wisdom, Snoop Dog!)

I'm not going to sugarcoat things: You may actually gain weight when working out. (I almost secretly hope you will, because it almost certainly means you are adding muscle.)

Now, that can trigger a lot of women because we are deeply brainwashed about a certain number we should be at to look good. What is it for you? 180? Under 150? Under 165? When my students start working out and building muscle, they almost always start to gain weight—and then they freak out and want to give up. Please, don't do that. Let's heal this together.

For starters, throw away the scale. The number on it has been linked to women's self-worth and well-being for far too long. It doesn't represent who you are, how magical your soul is, and what amazing things lie ahead of you once you break free from the mainstream starvation diets that keep you stressed and living in learned smallness—no matter what your physical size.

While writing this book, I took my mom on a retirement trip to the Maldives. We had so much time swimming in the warm Indian Ocean, playing sports, eating delicious fresh seafood, and being spoiled rotten. I watched my mom getting more and more relaxed while simultaneously being more energized and fuller of the life-force energy *chi*.

One evening, she remarked to me, "Wow, this swimsuit got so loose, I think I lost weight." She walked over to the scale in the hotel bathroom, pulled it out from underneath the sink, and weighed herself. My body started to tense. I had a flashback to my childhood and all those moments when my mom got onto the scale and dropped her shoulders in disappointment. "Not even one kilo less," she said. (We're European; we talk kilos to each other.)

"But, Mom, how do you feel?" I replied. "You look incredible! You seem to feel better." It didn't matter; she remained disappointed for the rest of the evening, even though she was physically in such a better place than she had been a week before.

Here's my point: We don't work out to lose weight; we work out for longevity, toning, anti-aging, managing glucose, posture, endorphins, and metabolic flexibility (that's the metaphor about switching between twigs and logs that we discussed earlier in the book). Please remember that this is about your health, not just (or even primarily) about your appearance.

Get Started

Why do I care so much about getting you moving? For starters, moving throughout the day helps you manage insulin (*Yay! We want that*), reduces your cortisol (*like a natural chill pill, so ...* hell yeah, *we want that*), and balances out hormones (*Damn straight, we want that, too*). The funny thing about working out is that it's hard to start, but once you make it a habit, you are addicted. For me, a day without movement feels awful. But I do remember the days when going to the gym felt intimidating, boring, and just plain unexciting.

Here's how I made the change.

F-I-T-N-E-S-S Framework

F: Frequency and Form

It's not enough to have one big two-hour workout once a week. It's much better to have shorter but more frequent workouts with multiple forms of movement throughout the day. As cliché as it sounds, take the stairs, work from a standing desk, and make an effort to stretch your legs every 40 to 60 minutes.

There was a study of 84 women who were cleaners for a living. The scientists told half of the group (the informed group) that their work was good exercise and counted as a great workout. The control group went on as usual with no feedback. Four weeks later, the women in the informed group lost weight, and their body mass index and blood pressure decreased, whereas the control group pretty much stayed the same.

What does it mean for you? Turn every household chore into a workout. Sweeping the floor? Imagine you just signed up for some elusive fad Hollywood personal trainer workout routine, and he's saying, "1, 2, 3, 4 to the left and 1, 2, 3, 4 to the right," along with some of your favorite jams. Laundry? Great, that's a workout, too; think of all the lifting and folding your arms are doing. Taking the trash out? *I'll do it, honey!* F is also for form because it's really important to do exercises correctly to avoid injuries and back issues.

I: Identity

Remember when I said that changing your identity is more powerful than "motivating yourself"? I can give you ten reasons why you should work out, but you probably know them already. But if I told you that, starting today, you are an athlete and athletes train, see how that feels in your body. Do you feel more purposeful and empowered? Fitness is who you are, not something that you do for an hour a day at the gym. The next time someone asks you why you train, tell them, "Because I'm an athlete. Duh!" And act accordingly.

T: Timing

Timing your workout with the natural way your hormones ebb and flow will make the workouts a whole lot easier and more effective. As women, we have both circadian and infradian rhythms, as we discussed above, so syncing your workout with your natural hormone fluctuations can be game changing. Certain hormones that aid in muscle recovery and growth, like testosterone and cortisol, peak in the morning, making it an optimal time for strength training and intense workouts, and now you know how to better match your workouts to your monthly cycle, too!

N: Nutrition

Food is fuel, but eating too close to a workout can leave you feeling sluggish, while not eating enough can result in a less effective training session. Timing your meals and snacks can drastically impact your workout performance and recovery (we will talk about it a little later), and we will look at the details of this in a moment. You want to make sure you replenish all the nutrients after a workout, especially protein; otherwise, you're just wearing out your body, not practicing fitness.

E: Enjoy and Endorphins

Remember, we don't do things that make us suffer. That's no longer wellness. Find a workout you enjoy and that gets you excited to leave the couch; later in the chapter, I'll mention a few I love, but the list is endless.

Also, endorphins—the happy hormones that get released when you move your body (otherwise known as "runner's high")—are the body's natural painkillers and mood elevators. Moving makes you feel good, and when you feel good, you go after your dreams. There is no amount of Tony Robbins that can get you out of a funk if you don't change your state and get moving. (Even Tony knows that!) Movement gets you happy and high for free, so why not use it?

S: Sweat

I hated sweating for years, but now I do everything I can to break a sweat at least once a day. Sweating flushes out toxins that you're bombarded with on a daily basis. It also fights germs, unclogs pores, and releases endorphins. Why spend money on fancy biohacking products when one of the best ones is free and always available?

S: Self

Self-esteem, self-confidence and self-respect. Fitness is a promise you make to yourself. It's between you and you. When you keep your own promise to yourself, you prove to yourself that you are important and that putting yourself first is not selfish. This is an act of self-kindness and a long-term investment in yourself and your health. It's not easy to show up at the gym or a class. Every time you do, you show your Higher Self that you can, which is great for building self-esteem, self-confidence, and self-respect—and this will translate into other areas of your life. You know you can count on you!

Walking

We are a generation of oversitters, overeaters, and overbreathers. According to the CDC, only 23% of Americans exercise regularly—and that doesn't mean going to the gym for a targeted workout; that means *any* kind of regular exercise.

What's the simplest way for many of us to make this change? Well, we all need to get places, right? And how are we going about doing that?

This is where I experienced the biggest culture shock when I moved from Europe to Los Angeles. No one seemed to walk anywhere.

Now, I understand that not everyone lives in urban areas where it's practical (or even possible) to walk to work or to the grocery store, but that doesn't mean you can't still find ways to squeeze in your steps. And speaking of which, do you really need 10,000 steps a day? Apparently not. A 2019 study published in *JAMA Internal Medicine* found that women who averaged around 4,400 steps per day had significantly lower mortality rates compared to women who took around 2,700 steps. The mortality rates progressively improved before leveling off at around 7,500 steps. Armed with this knowledge, I personally aim for at least 8,000 a day, and it's been great for my health. I usually hit that mark just going about my daily business, but it's not quite so high that I have to scramble at the end of the day to hit my goal.

And your walking doesn't have to be all practical walking to and from work, the store, or school. Walking, especially in nature, can enhance creative thinking. The combination of physical activity, relaxation, and a change in scenery can spur creative insights. But that's not all! In a recent interview, Dr. Andrew Huberman from Stanford University shared that the next time you feel anxiety, walk in an open space. Forward motion triggers the brain's "victory pathway," which is associated with bravery, courage, and audacity. It also allows you to snap out of tunnel vision (which can happen when you're stressed).

Movement Cancels Out Your Bio-Slacker Meal

There is an old Chinese saying, "散步走一走，活到九十九", which translates to "Take a walk after a meal, live to 99." This is a traditional practice based on the belief that taking a short walk after eating can aid digestion and overall well-being. (Side note: I am currently writing this in China, and yesterday my hosts suggested a quick walk around the city after our lunch, to the confusion of my American friends. So I can confirm that this practice is real.)

Modern research now proves this traditional Chinese saying to be true: *Moving after a meal helps lower our glucose.* (Read that again.) That means if you have a massive, carb-heavy dinner, go for a walk, vacuum, dance, or tidy up the house to help "cancel it out." Not only will this physical movement lower the stress retained in your body, but it's also a fast and sure way to burn up excess reserves of sugars in your bloodstream. And what does that do? Yup, you guessed it; it lowers your insulin levels!

If you can let go of stress and exercise with a positive mindset, any kind of activity can promote weight loss and better health. Think about all the activities that you do each day, and treat everything as if it is a part of your fitness routine. You'll be amazed at the positive changes you see.

Movement Hacks

Here are 20 ideas to weave more movement into the fabric of your daily routine:

1. Morning stretch: Begin your day with a five-minute stretch routine to wake up your muscles.

2. Deskercises: While at your desk, do seated leg lifts, desk push-ups, seated twists, or even simple fidgeting.

3. Walking meetings: Instead of sitting in a conference room, take your meetings outdoors and walk while you discuss. My girlfriends know I hate sitting for hours, and in Bali and LA, I always plan strategy sessions for beach walk meet-ups instead of coffee shops.

4. Take the stairs: Whenever you can, opt for stairs over the elevator.

5. Park further away: When shopping or at work, park your car farther from the entrance to add extra walking steps. They add up.

6. Dance breaks: Have a dance break every other hour while sitting at the desk. Put on your favorite song and dance hard for its entire duration.

7. Use a standing desk: Alternate between sitting and standing while working. I love my standing desk so much that I recently upgraded to a walking desk—a workstation on a treadmill.

8. Kitchen fitness: Do calf raises or squats while waiting for your food to cook.

9. SIT during TV ads: Get excited about a commercial break, don't skip it! Do a SIT workout (we will talk about that in a second) during commercial breaks or between episodes if you're streaming. Extra better if your partner or roommate can join!

10. Daily walks: Take a walk after meals, or dedicate a specific time each day for a walk, even if it's just 10-15 minutes.

11. Household chores: Vacuuming, gardening, and even washing dishes can be opportunities to move and stretch.

12. Cycle or walk errands: Instead of driving, consider walking or cycling for nearby errands.

13. Play with pets: If you have a dog, play fetch or take longer walks. Cats can also be engaged with toys that get both of you moving.

14. Be kind: Someone forgot something in the other room? I am the first one to offer "Let me get that for you" to get those extra steps! I get to burn extra calories *and* look like a selfless person. It's a win-win.

15. Take a new route: Change your usual walking or commuting path to keep things fresh.

16. Play with kids: If you have children or younger family members, play active games like tag or hide and seek.

17. Use fitness apps: Download the Cycle Bestie app that reminds you to move or guides you through short workouts.

18. Social activities: Instead of sedentary activities with friends, consider bowling, mini-golf, dancing, or hiking.

19. Volunteer: Participate in community service that requires movement, like helping in community gardens or organizing events.

20. Set reminders: Use your phone or computer to set hourly reminders encouraging you to stretch your legs or walk around for a few minutes.

Remember, it's not about the intensity or duration as much as it is about consistency. Every little bit of movement adds up throughout the day!

The Perfect Biohacking Workout: Work Out According to Your Cycle

If someone asks me what the best workout is for them, I always answer: It depends on which day of your cycle you're on! In the chapter about living according to your cycle, I told you which phases needed which type(s) of activity. Now, let me outline some of the different types of workouts you can choose from.

The next three workouts (HIIT, REHIT, and SIT training) not only *increase your metabolism* during the workout, but it stays elevated after the workout is complete, meaning your body is burning more calories at rest.

HIIT

High Intensity Interval Training (HIIT) typically involves exercises like sprints, burpees, or jump squats. Studies have shown that a 15-minute HIIT workout can burn more calories per minute than a 40-minute steady-state cardio workout.

Traditional HIIT consists of short bursts of intense exercise followed by brief recovery periods. For example, you go hard for 40 seconds and rest for 15. And then you repeat it for 15-20 minutes.

HIIT is great, but there is actually a better workout in town.

REHIT

What's even better than going hard for 40 seconds? Going full throttle, balls to the wall, as hard as you can for 15 to 20 seconds. You might be thinking, "Wait, how is that different?" The answer is, if you are able to "go hard" for a minute, this isn't actually your maximum capacity of 100%. Numerous studies have indicated that humans are able to give their absolutely max effort for only 15 to 20 seconds.

Now here is where REHIT gets even better. With HIIT, you rest for 15-20 seconds between exertion. With REHIT, you might rest anywhere between two and four minutes. The reason for this difference is that, while 15-20 seconds between workouts can be good for an athlete, most people (including myself) can't bring their heart rates back to their resting heart rate in such a short period of time. The longer rest period allows the heart rate to drop back toward a lower rate. Why does it matter? Because you want to be able to exercise your ability to go back to "homeostasis"—your resting state. Once your pulse is back to normal (around 60-75 beats per minute), you go all-out, absolutely maximum exertion for 15-20 seconds again, and you keep going as long as you can or for as much as your schedule allows.

SIT More

SIT (split interval training) is almost like running married REHIT training, and it's my favorite because I don't have to think of what exercise is next. While long-term running can place a lot of stress on joints and even be catabolic by burning muscle mass instead of fat, SIT is a great alternative.

How does it work? Sprint as hard as you can for 15-20 seconds, followed by recovery for as long as it takes to return your pulse to normal, and repeat as many times as you can. It is truly excellent for increasing fat burning. (Remember, we love our fat, but we also don't want to let it run the show.)

Weight Training

The same concept we discussed above for cardio workouts also applies to weight training. Rather than doing 50 reps with a light weight that doesn't push you to your maximum capacity, take those heavier weights (but be sure they aren't so heavy that they throw off your form or place unnecessary stress on your joints), and perform fewer but higher intensity repetitions until you have reached your maximum capacity. Follow this with—Yup! You guessed it: rest and recovery.

Gains in muscle strength are greatest when the weight load is greater, *not necessarily* when the repetitions are greater. The more intense weight overloads your muscles, which prompts them to add more cells in order to prevent this overload from happening again. (Your sympathetic nervous system kicks in with a fight or flight response, believing you're failing at something critical, like pushing off a bear or fighting a mountain lion!) Gradually increasing the weight forces your muscles into overload; this helps you continue to grow rather than allowing your body to grow accustomed to however much you're lifting and simply maintaining the same muscle mass.

Functional Training

Functional training workouts are one of my favorite types of workouts! These focus on movements that mimic real-life activities and improve overall functional fitness. They emphasize core stability, balance, coordination, and flexibility. Exercises may include squats, lunges, kettlebell swings, and medicine ball throws. Functional training workouts are usually my go-to around my period because they really complement that phase in my cycle well.

Pilates

Pilates is a low-impact exercise method that focuses on core strength, flexibility, and overall body conditioning. It involves controlled movements and emphasizes proper alignment and breathing techniques. Pilates exercises are often performed using specialized equipment or on a mat. My favorite is reformer Pilates (the machines are a bit different from the traditional form), and I always notice my muscles being super sore in places I didn't know existed!

Yoga

There are so many kinds of yoga, such as Hatha, Vinyasa, Ashtanga, Birham, Aero, and Yin—so before you say you don't like it, make sure you give each one a try to find your favorite. Yoga combines physical postures (*asanas*), breathing exercises, and meditation to promote flexibility, strength, balance, relaxation, and mental well-being. My favorite is hot yoga, which combines saunas and yoga. Through a lot of experimentation, I have found that Yin yoga at 8:30 p.m. in a heated room is profoundly spiritual and soothing for my body as I release the demands of the day and prepare my mind and body for sleep.

When to Work Out

When is the best time to work out? It depends, though your cortisol naturally rises in the morning, so you could use this as an extra burst of energy during your workout.

Also, "To eat or not to eat before a morning workout?" That is the question I get a lot. The short answer is (again): it depends. In this case, it depends on what your goal is!

Fasted Versus Non-Fasted Workouts

There is a lot of conflicting advice on whether to work out while fasting or not fasting. Some research shows that exercising while in a fasted state will place your body into more ketosis and also efficiently burn fat because you have already eliminated a lot of the glycogen stores in your muscles and liver.

However, exercising is, as we've discussed, a stressor on the body, and so is fasting. So what happens when you combine two stressors (or add the third one: phase 4 of your cycle)? *No bueno.* The key here is balance. Exercising in a fasted state every day might be a case of too much of a good thing. On days where you feel as though you have been well rested in the period leading up to exercise, with relatively low exposure to other stressors, an exercise session in a fasted state will be productive and not throw your body (or its cortisol levels) into disarray.

Importantly as well, a nutrient-rich meal of fats, protein, and fiber (rather than sugar- or artificial sweetener-filled shakes or sugary pre-workout snacks) is essential for refueling your body after a fasted state to avoid placing it in a high-glucose, high-insulin state of stress.

My rule of thumb is this: fasted workouts are okay for lighter workouts; save weight-lifting for after breakfast. We will talk about managing stress more in our dedicated chapter on stress, but by now, you should be seeing all the wonderful moving parts of biohacking coming together to show you the flexibility, control, and freedom that it offers when you take ownership of your body and biohack into strength, wellness, and efficiency.

3x3 Micro-Workouts

We had micro-fasts, and now we have ... micro-workouts! Remember at the very start when I said that fitness is who you are, not what you do? Well, instead of putting aside an hour a day to work out and then failing to follow through, plan three 3-minute workouts right before a meal. Remember, you can turbocharge your fat-burning abilities if you work out when you feel the first signs of hunger. So before breakfast, lunch, and dinner (maybe even as the food is cooking, if you can make that work) do some high knees or burpees for 20-30 seconds. Repeat three times and enjoy your meal!

Recovery & Stretching

Oversitting is bad for you, but so is overtraining. I am a big believer in the idea that we want to *work* out, not *wear* out, our bodies. Ensure that your body has enough time to recover. Not recovering places it into a state of chronic stress which elevates hormones such as corti-sol, which in turn promotes increased fat storage over fat burning. So with HIIT/REHIT/SIT and weight training, rest and recovery go hand-in-hand—not only during the exercises but after them, too.

I personally don't like stretching, but after skydiving for a few days, followed by three days of mountain biking in Switzerland, followed by a 16-hour flight to New York City, I could barely move for a week. My lower back was in so much pain I couldn't stand or sit. What did my acupuncturist say when I went in for a treatment? *Did you stretch at all?* Of course I didn't. I was "too busy," and stretching was boring because sometimes I turn back into a twelve-year-old and think I'm too cool to do basic human things. You would think that I learned something during that stiff, painful week in NYC, but no. It took another few months and more lower back pains to realize that maybe I should stop thinking that I could somehow magically bypass the need to prepare my muscles for intense physical activity and actually, you know, *prepare my muscles for intense physical activity.*

Stretching is now my go-to before I work out. It's amazing how much better I feel immediately afterward, as well as during my recovery periods, when I actually do the thing I'm supposed to do. Stretch-ing doesn't have to be a whole thing; just spend a few minutes gen-tly moving, bending, and generally just warming up your muscles before you begin a workout.

Which would you rather have: a friend texts you to ask if you'd like to work out together and to be ready when she swings by in ten minutes? Or a friend wakes you up by standing over your bed with a bullhorn, screaming, "GET UP! WE'RE GOING TO SPRINT A MARATHON RIGHT NOW!" Be a good friend to yourself.

And please remember that recovery is equally important. I do all kinds of movement every day, but you want to take your rest days as seriously as the workout days. I follow a lot of extra-ripped male fitness influencers running 10 miles every morning after lifting weights for an hour, and I want to do the same. Well, I mean, I *want* to want to do the same because, hey, it's working for them, right? But I also want to respect my body, and when I've promised her a down day to repair herself so that she is ready for the next workout, I think I owe it to her to honor that commitment.

Overtraining is actually more problematic for women than under-training, especially around your period. There is something called the Female Athlete Triad syndrome which is often seen in physically active girls and women, and it involves three interconnected conditions: 1) low energy due to not eating enough calories, 2) hormonal imbalance (lack or irregular period), and 3) low bone density.

Wrap Up

The most important thing that you can take from this chapter is the mindset that we are working toward *health first*. Getting skinny, getting jacked, being "hardcore" — none of that stuff means that you are healthy. If your only motivation for biohacking is to look a certain way, you are almost certainly going to end up doing things to your body that cause more damage than good.

Of course, I want you to love the way you look, but it's more important to me that you love the way you *feel*. If you follow the suggestions I'm offering here, you will absolutely start to see positive changes in your body, but those are just the cherry on top of the thriving, nourished, gorgeous sundae you've created through thoughtful workouts and mindful eating. (Yeah, I know. I started that sentence, and then it didn't really work all the way to the end, but I'd already committed to it, so . . . well, we give ourselves grace in all things. Even bad metaphors.)

KEY TAKEAWAYS

- **Focus on Health, Not Just Size:** Shift the emphasis from achieving a certain weight to building strength and muscle for a healthier body composition.

- **Tailor Workouts to Menstrual Cycle:** Adapt your exercise routine to align with the different phases of your menstrual cycle, utilizing workouts like HIIT, REHIT, and SIT for their unique benefits.

- **Embrace Micro-Workouts:** Incorporate short and frequent workouts into your daily activities, making fitness more practical and manageable.

- **Balance Fasted and Fed Workouts:** Consider the type of workout and your body's needs when choosing to exercise in a fasted state or after eating.

- **Prioritize Recovery and Stretching:** Recognize the importance of rest, recovery, and stretching as essential components of a well-rounded fitness regimen.

CHAPTER 8

SLEEP WELL

"Does it even count as 'sleeping with him' if I didn't get any REM sleep?"

—my biohacker friend, after a date night

We all know that one person who is constantly pushing, hustling, and going a million miles an hour, 24/7. We may even admire her "Sleep when you're dead" spirit.

But the thing is, we're all going to die a lot sooner—or at least set ourselves up for a chronic illness—if we adopt that mentality. Think about it, in extreme conditions, you can go almost a month without food, almost a week without water, but only days without sleep. Only oxygen beats sleep in terms of things your body needs to survive.

Biohackers are obsessed with sleep, and I hope you will be soon, too. A lot of my students are young moms who immediately want to skip over this part. "Aggie, I have two under two," I hear. "I don't have nine hours in a day to stay in bed." I get it; that's real. And that is also why we need to make you a sleep ninja so that you make sure that each second of your sleep matters. To you, my bestie without enough hours in the day, this chapter is *especially* for you!

Bryan Johnson is a biohacker who spends $2 million a year "trying not to die" (his words) by trying all the tech and treatments on the planet to reverse his biological age (which is now much less than his chronological age). He also had a six-month streak of hitting a perfect sleep score on one of the popular wearable devices, giving him the title of the best sleeper in history. Want to guess what Bryan's #1 anti-aging tip is? Yup: sleep!

He says he's not motivated to work out, eat well, or even be nice to himself when he doesn't hit his perfect 100% sleep score. He describes the life of getting great sleep as magical.

Are you surprised you struggle with sticking to eating healthy or being kind to your partner when you're operating in a chronic sleep deficit?

Most of us (I take that back), *all* of us—myself included, don't get anywhere near Bryan's sleep score. If you are a mom, live in a city, or have this pesky thing called *real life* going on, I am pretty sure you could use some better sleep.

But why does our sleep collectively suck as a society? Because we are surrounded by artificial light, electronics, electromagnetic fields (EMFs), hot bedrooms, and late dinners (Bryan has his dinner at noon! That's a little extreme if you ask me, but it clearly works for him).

Even though, from an evolutionary perspective, sleep doesn't make any sense, because why would you spend a third of your life in a vulnerable state where you can't do much? But scientists are slowly starting to understand why we get smarter, fitter, and kinder when we get enough sleep.

Sleep really needs to become a viral TikTok trend; maybe then everyone would start getting what they need. Imagine a world in which "Hey, sorry I'm late, I just needed to sleep longer today" is a valid excuse to miss a meeting, and the response is, "Of course! Take any time you need."

Instead, we live in a world where sleeping until your body is sated is looked down on as a sign of laziness, and your friends call you "Grandma" when you suggest a 4 p.m. dinner because you want it to settle before going to bed. (Ask me how I know.)

When your body and mind are rested, you tend to see things very differently than when your energy is depleted. With good sleep, you probably look around and feel more expansive, and see the world as more supportive, friendly, and full of opportunities. Even your immune system is better off. Let's face it, sleep is pretty much the superhero of health. Without it, you're not just tired, you're setting yourself up for a domino effect that can knock down your health, productivity, and well-being.

When you improve your sleep quality, several positive changes occur:

Weight loss becomes easier. A lack of sleep disrupts your body's ability to know when you're full. Sleep increases leptin, an appetite suppressant, and decreases ghrelin, an appetite stimulant. Poor sleep flips this, leading to increased hunger. If you find yourself raiding the fridge late at night, it might be due to insufficient sleep.

We grow muscle faster. Sleep is crucial for recovery and muscle growth, as the body produces growth hormones predominantly during sleep. These hormones repair tissues and aid in muscle development. Athletes often need about eight hours of sleep for optimal recovery and performance improvement. As someone who is now embracing her identity as an athlete and wanting to grow muscle, this should be great news for you.

We become better at emotions. Better sleep leads to less reactivity and better emotional processing, which positively affects your relationships. This is why the old advice to "sleep on it" is so wise!

We manage blood sugar better. Insufficient sleep can cause your blood sugar levels to rise, even in response to healthy foods. While it might sound like something out of a sci-fi book, it's true; a lack of sleep can lead to unexpected blood sugar spikes, leading to increased sugar cravings.

We're more productive. Contrary to the belief that all-nighters are productive, quality sleep actually enhances concentration, productivity, and problem-solving abilities. Also, tasks often expand to fill the time allotted for them, so it's more efficient to set shorter deadlines and ensure good sleep.

We stress less. Adequate sleep each night plays a key role in managing stress. It can also alleviate anxiety, depression, and other mental health issues related to stress. Quality sleep is a cornerstone of good mental health.

Sleep Disruptors

So why is our sleep so poor? If this was a Marvel movie, Sleep would be reigning over the world until Thomas Edison invented artificial light, and then our bodies got completely confused, and sleep started being considered unnecessary and anti-capitalistic.

My life is split between Bali and Los Angeles, and I travel 300 days a year. With constant time zone changes, I struggle to get good sleep, and the main reason is light! When it comes to sleep, light is a (if not *the*) game changer. Let me explain with a bit of my jet-setting life as an example.

Imagine this: I land in Bali, and it's 17 hours ahead of the U.S. My body clock is screaming, "It's 11 a.m." because it is … in Los Angeles. But in Bali, it's 3 a.m. I'm only running on five hours of sleep, but here I am, wide awake, even though everyone in Bali is fast asleep. That's my circadian rhythm at play. It's like an internal conductor, orchestrating the release of hormones like melatonin, the sleep hormone we touched on in the hormone chapter.

Here's where light comes into play, and it's not just a factor when jet lag and hopping time zones are in the mix. Light affects our sleep *daily*. Our modern lives are swamped with artificial lights like phones, lamps, TVs, and even streetlights. These are the sneaky culprits that mess with our circadian rhythm.

When I'm trying to combat jet lag, or just trying to get a good night's sleep in my own bed, managing light exposure is key. Whether I've just flown to Bali or I'm waking up on a regular Tuesday in LA, I try to expose myself to natural light first thing in the morning. It's like sending a signal to my brain, recalibrating it to the local time. That might mean waiting a few hours for the sun to come up once I've landed somewhere, but I would rather do that than pull all the shades in my room and sleep until noon. I also avoid bright screens and harsh lights before bedtime—which is always a good idea, but *especially* when I'm traveling and know my time zones are a bit scrambled. It's all about mimicking the natural light-dark cycle, and telling our bodies when it's time to wind down and time to amp up.

Whether it's fighting off jet lag or just catching some quality Zzzs in our hectic lives, remember: light is more than just brightness. It's the natural cue that sets our sleep rhythms. But it's not the only factor.

Would you be surprised to learn that alcohol is actually one of the biggest sleep disruptors? I have heard so many women say that they like to have a glass or two of wine in the evenings to relax and help them sleep. While this may be okay, heavier alcohol consumption will keep you in a lighter sleep, so you don't get the beneficial REM cycle.

Caffeine is another culprit. While caffeine is great for waking us up in the morning, if we have a coffee in the afternoon, half of it will still be in our bodies by midnight! Along with coffee, caffeine is also present in colas, chocolate, and certain teas (black and green are particularly high). Each body metabolizes caffeine differently, but a good gauge of when to cut off caffeine in the day is usually by 1-2 p.m., and keep in mind that the body's ability to metabolize caffeine tends to slow as we age. So while an afternoon cappuccino may have quickly cleared your system when you were 18, at age 30, it might take a lot longer.

Also, adding to the many other reasons to stop smoking, nicotine is a stimulant that can cause users to have lighter sleep during the night and wake up too early because their body is going through nicotine withdrawal.

Finally, even something as seemingly innocuous as eating a large meal late at night can mess with your gut by causing indigestion, which could keep you awake. And remember our conversation about "too much of a good thing"? Drinking too much fluid right before sleep can cause you to keep waking up to make those repeated trips to the bathroom, disrupting your sleep cycles. So guzzle your water, but lay off a bit about 60-90 minutes before bedtime.

Measuring Sleep

While the amount of sleep you get can be a good indicator that you are sleeping enough, the *quality of sleep* you're getting is an important factor, too. Sleep trackers can come in handy for monitoring your sleep. I use an Oura ring, which can help track how long I am staying in each cycle or type of sleep, whether my heart rate is high or low, and how long it takes to fall asleep. Ideally, you want to aim for 7-9 hours a night with at least 90 minutes of REM and 90 minutes of deep sleep. That's why it's important to measure. You can get eight straight hours of sleep, but only 20-30 minutes of deep sleep (which is very common after a night out), and then be confused about why you're so tired the next day.

An example of a bad night's sleep and a good night's sleep using my Oura ring.

Sleep Cycles

Your nights are composed of recurring sleep stages, including phases of light sleep, deep sleep, and REM sleep. Light sleep makes up about half of your time in dreamland, and (ideally), the other half is made up of 50% REM and 50% deep sleep.

During light sleep, your breathing and heart rate both slow, but the brain has periodic bursts of electrical activity that are believed to help with sorting information taken in during the day to allow you to learn and retain the more important information while weeding out the less significant things.

"REM," short for Rapid Eye Movement, describes the rapid side-to-side eye movements during this sleep phase. While dreams are most commonly associated with REM sleep, they can occur at other times, too. This stage is crucial for emotional processing, memory retention, and creativity. Many sleep scientists consider REM the most important stage of the sleep cycle for cognitive function during our waking hours. A deficit in REM sleep can leave you feeling tired, moody, and stressed upon waking.

Deep sleep, or slow-wave sleep (SWS) is a restorative phase where the body conducts internal housekeeping: healing organs, reducing blood pressure, detoxifying, repairing muscles, and processing glucose. During SWS, the brain exhibits delta wave patterns, indicative of deep, non-REM sleep. This stage is vital for physical and mental rejuvenation, marked by a significant release of growth hormone, which fosters tissue repair and cognitive enhancement. SWS also engages the parasympathetic nervous system, reducing stress responses and promoting cardiovascular health through lowered heart and respiratory rates. This deep sleep predominantly occurs in the early part of the night, while REM sleep increases closer to the morning.

There is one other type of rest that you should be aware of, however, and that is non-sleep deep rest (NSDR), which operates by slowing down brain waves, similar to what occurs during a restorative, or SWS sleep. NSDR mirrors these effects, transitioning brain wave frequencies from the alert beta state, through the relaxed alpha, to the theta state of deep meditation. Remarkably, NSDR can even evoke delta frequencies, typically exclusive to SWS, which allows it to replicate the restorative benefits of deep sleep *while you remain awake.*

This is particularly beneficial since many people do not consistently achieve SWS during their nightly sleep.

NSDR aids in memory retention, enhances neuroplasticity for improved learning, relieves stress, boosts cognitive function, and can even help with pain management. To engage in NSDR, you can practice yoga nidra, and hypnosis. Yoga nidra is a guided meditation that leads to a state between wakefulness and sleep, aiding in relaxation and reaching that deep stage of rest—especially if your body struggles to reach it during regular sleep.

Alternatively, hypnosis induces a trance-like state of deep focus and relaxation, useful for addressing anxiety, stress, and mood disorders. Both methods require discipline and dedicated practice in a distraction-free environment, but they can offer a pathway to experience the profound benefits of deep rest separate from sleep.

Sleep Chronotypes

You don't need to be a morning person to get good sleep, even though we morning people definitely are annoying at making every other chronotype feel bad for not waking up at 5 a.m. (Sorry about that.) Everyone has a personal sleep chronotype, which affects their peak functioning times, so if you don't love mornings, don't worry. Sleep chronotypes fall into three groups: early risers, night owls, and those who fall in between the two.

Early risers, or morning chronotypes, are energized in the early hours and most productive at the start of the day; they generally fall asleep soon after dusk and naturally wake up just before sunrise.

Evening chronotypes, or night owls, are more inclined to wake up later and feel more active in the afternoon and evening hours; they tend to wake up later and continue working well past sundown.

If you're the third intermediate chronotype, you have some flexibility in your sleep and wake times. You might not feel exceptionally bright and chipper first thing in the morning, nor do you feel your best late at night. Instead, your peak times are somewhere in the middle of the day.

Each of us operates on a circadian rhythm, that 24-hour internal clock that cycles between alertness and sleepiness that we discussed earlier. Also known as the sleep/wake cycle, this rhythm is unique to each person. Understanding and aligning with your natural circadian rhythm is essential, as ignoring it can negatively affect your overall well-being. (Keep in mind, though, that your chronotype is not set in stone; you can actually shift your type by setting new habits either by intentionally cultivating different practices or unintentionally simply by repeated behaviors.)

How to Biohack Your Sleep

Let me say it again for the people in the back: *sleep is the easiest, cheapest, and best biohack.* Learning how to master it can be crucial to your progress.

First, create your sleep sanctuary. Prioritize a bedroom that's cool, dark, and quiet. A slightly cooler bedroom temperature can facilitate the body's natural drop in core temperature, which aids in sleep. Black-out curtains are a must, as well as turning off all electronics in the room that emit blue light. If you ever share a hotel room with me, you'll see me maniacally covering air-conditioning lighting with a towel or the red light on the TV with a tissue box – anything that prevents total darkness. Also, any overhead light will confuse your sleep-wake cycle, so use bedside lamps or anything below your eye line.

Get your phone onboard. When it comes to your phone, there is a "black and white" setting on the iPhone that you can set to switch on automatically past sunset. It makes sitting on your phone scrolling through cat videos so much less appealing. There is also a filter that you can set to reduce the amount of blue light put out by your screen after sundown.

Set a regular sleep schedule. Consistency is key. Unfortunately, undersleeping during the week only to sleep in on weekends is not going to work. Try to go to sleep and wake up at a similar time to give your body the predictability it needs.

Pay attention to your diet and sleep. Be mindful of caffeine and alcohol intake, especially close to bedtime. Avoid large meals late at night.

Maximize morning light for better sleep. Expose yourself to natural light within 20 minutes of waking up. It signals your brain to wake up and aligns your circadian rhythm. Dim lights and minimize screen time in the evening. This helps prepare your body for sleep by increasing natural melatonin production.

Engage in daily physical activity. Regular exercise, preferably not close to bedtime, can significantly improve sleep quality. If you want to move your body closer to bedtime, I love pre-sleeping walks with Peanut Butter, my dog.

Utilize naps judiciously. A short, 20-minute nap in the afternoon can be rejuvenating. However, avoid longer naps that can disrupt your nighttime sleep routine.

Set your alarm for 9 p.m.(!), not a.m. Really! I tell my students that, just as you set an alarm to wake up, set one for bedtime to start your pre-sleep routine. It allows you to have more time to get ready for sleep—maybe to take a warm bath or shower or to spend a little time with infrared therapy before curling up in bed.

When I am deep into another Netflix show and my alarm goes off, I take it as seriously as a morning alarm—no snoozing, no "Just a few more minutes." And now, (I know you're going to hate me for this, and I'm sorry, but) I actually never set a morning alarm anymore. I wake up naturally between 6 and 6:30 a.m. every morning, fully rested and ready to take on a new day.

If you can't fall asleep, I recommend anything that helps you unwind: journaling, boxed breathwork, or even bedtime stories. (Who said we grew out of them?)

Also, keep in mind that sleep quality can change during different phases of your cycle. It may be more difficult to fall asleep or stay asleep in the luteal (post-ovulatory) phase of your cycle because of your shifting hormones. The more aware you are of your body's rhythms through living according to your cycle, the better prepared you can be for this monthly shift, and you can be prepared to adapt accordingly.

Remember, sleep is great. Even if you aren't a sleep-overachiever like Bryan Johnson, you can still take certain steps that allow you to use the one-third of your life that you aren't conscious to your advantage.

You may not ever love mornings, and that's okay. But maybe with some intentionality, you can at least learn to hate them less, and maybe that's progress.

KEY TAKEAWAYS

- **Sleep—A Non-Negotiable Health Pillar:** Sleep is crucial for survival, surpassing the need for food and water in the short term. Good sleep leads to improved mental, physical, and emotional health.

- **Light Management for Better Sleep:** Managing light exposure, both natural and artificial, are important to regulate the circadian rhythm and enhance sleep quality.

- **Impact of Diet and Lifestyle on Sleep:** Alcohol, caffeine, and late-night eating can disrupt sleep. Advocate for mindful eating and drinking habits to support better sleep.

- **Power of Sleep Tracking and Understanding Cycles:** Encourage the use of sleep trackers to monitor sleep quality and understand the different sleep stages (light sleep, REM, deep sleep) for overall well-being.

- **Personalize Your Sleep Strategy:** Tailor sleep practices to your individual needs, including recognizing your sleep chronotype and creating a conducive sleep environment. Highlight the role of physical activity and pre-sleep routines in improving sleep quality.

CHAPTER 9

STRESS

"You're not doing too much, you're doing too little that sets your soul on fire."

—Aggie Lal

I don't remember where I first heard these two quotes, but they have stayed with me for years. I try to incorporate them in the personal coaching I do, as well, because I have seen firsthand how this profound wisdom can be life-changing.

Take, for example, Molly. Molly tried every biohack on the planet. She adjusted her diet based on her DNA, she scheduled intense workouts with the best personal trainers, she fasted like an absolute champ—and yet she saw no results. "Is biohacking a scam?" she finally asked me in despair one day. "What else can I do?"

I looked at her schedule, filled to the brim with work demands and biohacks, and the problem immediately became apparent. "Molly, do less," I told her, "not more." We scheduled an hour of *dolce far niente* for her ("the sweetness of doing nothing" in Italian, because Italians get it!). No phone. No working out. Just an hour outside, walking, looking off in the distance—not doing, just being. We discussed the importance of making this a regular practice in her life.

A month later, Molly messaged me: "Aggie, I lost 15 lbs. How is that possible? I did nothing!"

Exactly. She was overworked and overtrained. High cortisol was making her hold on to belly fat, made her crave salty and sugary foods, and kept her bloated and miserable. It's about the Goldilocks rule: Not too much, not too little—juuuuust right.

Look, I'm not a fortune teller, but let me guess: You also feel a little too much stress in your life? And I'm not even talking about Bob from accounting making a sexist remark and pissing you off (though that's real, and I'm sorry you have to deal with that jackass on the daily). I'm talking in general. You have gotten so resilient at kicking ass while being tired and sleep deprived that you don't even notice how depleted you are until you take away your coffee and a phone for a few hours. Suddenly, your exhaustion and overcommitment both become crystal clear.

Stress has infiltrated our body's biology like a spy so thoroughly that it's no longer just a fleeting visitor, like the pounding heart we experience in a near-miss on the road. Stress doesn't come and go anymore; now, it's more like background noise that never quite fades, a persistent hum that underlies every moment, much like the ceaseless buzz of electricity in a city that never sleeps. It's omnipresent, seeping into the nooks and crannies of our day, a subtle but constant whisper reminding us of the endless "what ifs" and "should haves" and "must dos" until those become the soundtrack of our everyday lives.

While we are very good at acute (short-term) stress that helps us either fight, run away, or freeze when attacked by a tiger, nature hasn't prepared us for chronic (prolonged) stress. Yet that is the condition in which we are living day in and day out in our modern world.

We are so accustomed to chronic stress and so resilient that it's really hard to tell if we are actually stressed or not. Our baseline is *that* screwed up. Our autonomic nervous system (ANS) encompasses two main branches: the sympathetic nervous system, which orchestrates the "fight or flight" response during perceived danger or stress, and the parasympathetic nervous system, which promotes the "rest and digest" (which I like to call "rest and receive") activities that occur when the body is at rest.

It's quite easy to tell if you're acutely, actively stressed. Even though I have done over 300 skydives, I still experience a typical fight-or-flight response as I am standing on the verge of a plane with my parachute on: increased heart rate, sweating, dry mouth, adrenaline rush, and needing to pee. And they all go away the moment I open my parachute.

But what about chronic stress? Chronic, prolonged stress is when your body produces high levels of cortisol for long periods of time, such as when you feel overwhelmed and pressured by things in your life, and you live in that space until it sometimes almost begins to feel normal.

Chronic stress is way more subtle. Maybe it takes you hours to get out of bed and get going so you think you're not a morning person. You need an obscene amount of coffee to get up and running, yet you are awake in the evenings, zoning out and trying to numb your feelings by scrolling through another makeup tutorial on TikTok.

Maybe you struggle with bloating, indigestion, GERD, or migraines. Maybe you're tired all the time or anxious. Or maybe you get colds all the time or wake up to pee five times during the night. Or maybe you just have no patience when your friend Kate takes 20 minutes to share with you another dating story she has that you know is going to end in the exact same way, with the guy being nowhere near good enough for her, but her wondering if "Maybe there's some potential there?" Or maybe you struggle to want to have sex or even just be around other humans.

These persistent high levels of cortisol can lead to chronic fatigue, which results in our bodies storing fat, especially around our belly. High cortisol also impacts glucose. Being stressed is almost like having an extra Oreo every day, even though you stick to eating salads only. It's like an "on" switch to long-term health issues that are usually dormant and manifest after prolonged periods of stress.

Can you measure stress? Yes. Just as a CGM (Continuous Glucose Monitor) measures your glucose, different wearables like the Oura Ring track your HRV (heart rate variability), which is the space between your heartbeats. There is no right number; however, the lower the HRV, the more stressed your body tends to be.

If you do nothing about managing your stress, your cortisol may begin rising and falling at the wrong times during the day, leaving you feeling groggy in the morning and wide awake at night. With chronic fatigue, your cortisol is low all the time, leaving you feeling exhausted no matter how much sleep you get. You might find yourself becoming more and more dependent on those cups of coffee to get you through the day.

High levels can also activate certain diseases that may run in your family. If you have a genetic predisposition for certain conditions that are otherwise lying dormant, these increased levels could turn on those genes. (This is the study of epigenetics: how your behaviors and environment can cause changes that affect your genes, which is a whole other topic for a whole other time. But it's real, and it's absolutely worth considering when we talk about the long-term impact of chronic stress.)

How to Deal With Stress

There are many different ways to deal with stress. The first one would be: stress less. I know, I know. That's about as helpful as telling someone "Calm down." Or "Just chill." Or "Don't sweat the small stuff." Or, "Geez, why can't you relax?"

OMG, are you annoyed yet? Just look at all the different ways that society has figured out how to tell us to ignore our feelings because we are being "too emotional" or making things more complicated than they need to be. Do you know what that does? *It just makes us more stressed.* The thing is, stress doesn't live in our heads, it lives in our bodies. It's our bodies that carry the weight and bear the signs of all this stress, so we want to make sure we biohack it where it happens. We need body-related techniques to help us remove it—not just "thinking happy thoughts."

Heal Stress With a Sigh

The best real-time solution is alerting your breath. This isn't exactly breathwork, which we will talk about a little later; this is biohacking your diaphragm to engage your parasympathetic nervous system.

There are two ways to do this. One is to make your exhale longer than your inhale. For example, inhale for three seconds and exhale for six.

Or you can practice a physiological sigh, which is a specific breathing technique that has been identified by neuroscientists like Dr. Andrew Huberman, a neuroscientist at Stanford University, as a natural and effective way to regulate stress and emotional responses. This breathing pattern is something we often do unconsciously, particularly when we're feeling relieved or comforted—for example after a good cry or right before we're about to fall asleep.

The physiological sigh consists of a double inhalation followed by a longer, slower exhalation. Here's how it works:

First inhale: Take a deep breath in through your nose.

Second inhale: Before exhaling, take another small inhale on top of the first one. This is typically a shorter, quicker breath.

Exhale: Finally, exhale slowly through your mouth, ideally making the exhale longer than the combined inhales.

The purpose of this breathing pattern is to rapidly re-oxygenate the body and, more effectively, to expel carbon dioxide. The double inhale helps to reinflate any alveoli—tiny air sacs in the lungs—that may have collapsed during shallow breathing, which is common during states of stress. The longer exhale then aids in the removal of carbon dioxide and triggers the body's relaxation response.

Heal Stress With ... More Stress

There are so many biohacks to help you lower your stress on a daily basis. The key is to find the ones that speak to you so that you will incorporate them into your routine. Some of them actually heal stress with more stress. Really! That's because not all stress is bad for us.

There is a type of stress called hormetic stress, which is a long-lost cousin of the chronic stress we want to get rid of. Hormetic stress is stress that challenges us—pushes us just a bit, like a motivational coach—but doesn't exhaust us or break us down. It puts us in a very stressful situation for a short period of time and exercises our ability to come back to homeostasis—a state where we belong.

Hormetic stress is good for you in small doses because it makes you realize your potential and builds up your sense of accomplishment and confidence. It helps you lose weight, become stronger, and look younger. Some examples of this could include cold therapy, such as ice baths or cold showers, which are great for stress management.

Small Stuff Isn't Small—It's Trauma

Now, let's talk about chronic stress. A lot of chronic stress comes from the trauma we experience as children that continues to replay in our adult life. Your body "keeps the score," as the popular expression goes. It remembers stressful situations from the past and childhood, and any reminder triggers a stress response.

What doctors used to think of as trauma is war, natural disaster, physical assault, or serious accident, which can then lead to PTSD. But most of us experience trauma without ever going to war. Today, experts like Dr. Gabor Maté, a renowned physician and author of *The Myth of Normal*, and Dr. Bessel van der Kolk, the author of the aptly-named *The Body Keeps the Score*, realize that this definition is incomplete and have worked to redefine the popular understanding of trauma.

Maté defines trauma as "any experience that overwhelms our capacity to cope and leaves us feeling helpless, powerless, and out of control. Trauma is not just about the bad things that might have happened to you; it can occur as a result of what didn't happen (like not being seen, heard, or understood)."

He argues that trauma happens when we are left in a seemingly small event without emotional support and connection from our caregivers. Then, years later, when we are in a somewhat similar experience, we tend to have a disproportionate reaction to a seemingly small event because it uproots a bigger trauma that hasn't healed.

What's really common is to spiritually bypass our not-so-hard experiences with dismissive thoughts like "Well, others have it worse" or "How can you stress about work when others have no food to eat."

Unfortunately, not acknowledging our own real-life challenges and our own capacity to cope makes that experience even worse.

Unexpressed Feelings Create Stress

The idea of "spiritual bypassing" refers to the process of glossing over difficult experiences with comparisons or platitudes that diminish the validity of our own pain. It's a kind of avoidance that ignores the real and often necessary process of confronting and working through our emotions.

Take Alex, who, as a child, often tried to share her accomplishments with her parents. Whenever she did, her parents were either too busy or simply not interested. They never acknowledged her efforts or celebrated her successes, leading her to feel ignored and unimportant.

Fast forward to Alex's adult life. In her workplace, when her contributions are overlooked, or her colleagues don't listen to her during meetings, she experiences an intense emotional reaction. Her boss not noticing her efforts could lead to chronic stress at work. From the outside, these current experiences trigger feelings of inadequacy and invisibility rooted in her childhood. The original trauma wasn't a single, life-threatening event, but it was a series of moments where the lack of attention made her feel undervalued and unsupported. This reaction is not just about the present moment of being ignored; it's amplified by a history of similar experiences. Comparing her situation to those in more dire circumstances (What about children starving in the developing world? Your childhood was amazing by comparison; what do you have to complain about?) invalidates her feelings and can exacerbate the distress.

The "what-about-ism" is actually a propaganda technique used to dismiss someone's point or pain. You can deeply care about starving children *and* feel deeply upset about Lauren in HR saying something snide about you at work. You can be both grateful to have children *and* miss your single life. You can love your husband *and* know you deserve better. You can love your body and want to biohack to feel even better. You have the right to feel what you feel, even if it's conflicting at times. Suppressing difficult emotions with toxic gratitude is not doing anyone a favor.

By acknowledging the deep-seated feelings, you can begin to understand your triggers and work toward healing the trauma that arises from patterns of repeated hurtful behavior. And that's how we change this planet for the better: Not by one-upping each other with our trauma and hardship, but by acknowledging it's a reality in so many lives and then doing the work to heal it.

Feel It to Heal It

Which gender is more culturally programmed to suppress healthy anger and to serve as the "peacemakers" and "caregivers"? Women, of course.

Likewise, which gender, according to the American Autoimmune Related Diseases Association (AARDA), accounts for 80% of autoimmune disease patients in the United States? Women again. Conditions like lupus, rheumatoid arthritis, chronic fatigue, fibromyalgia disease, Hashimoto syndrome, and inflammatory disease of the gut are all markedly higher in women than any other gender. Is there a connection between unexpressed emotions like anger and resentment and the immune system attacking its own body?

There are many theories, but Dr. Maté's trauma research has led him to conclude that women get sick from unprocessed emotions. We women tend to be hyperaware about the emotional needs of others, rather than our own. We tend to suppress healthy anger because we are trained to be "good girls." We also tend to believe that we are responsible for how other people feel and that we must never disappoint anybody—"Two fatal beliefs," Maté says. According to research, the "thoughtful, nice girls" (is this you?) are more likely to develop immune diseases than women who don't put others' needs before their own.

Heal Stress With Being a Bitch

If there is one thing I truly believe, it's that none of the biohacking will work if we don't take care of and learn to healthily express our emotions. Every disease is a manifestation of a dis-ease in our body, including (especially?) emotional triggers. We've all been there. A sucky break-up that leaves you with a runny nose. Getting ill when going on holidays with the family or coming back from a trip to visit relatives.

We're often boxed into roles of being endlessly sweet and consider-ate—afraid to ruffle feathers or cause disappointment. But let's face it, we're not responsible for managing everyone's emotions. You can't possibly "make someone angry." Adults are responsible for their emotions.

Striving to always be "the better person" can be a suffocating cage. Women often feel like we need to be sweet and considerate, and never hurt anyone's feelings or offend them. I get it; I've lived this exhausting reality, too. Wanting so hard to be liked by everyone caused me to lose a lot of time, inner peace, and, above all, myself.

Society often has a harsh label for women who dare to say no, who prioritize themselves; they're quickly branded as "bitches." That label triggered and stung the hell out of me at first. I bent over back-ward to avoid disappointing anyone: my followers, my family, my friends, and my significant others.

But then, after exploring Dr. Gabor Maté and Dr. Bessel van der Kolk's work on trauma and delving into the world of biohacking, a realization struck. Many women deal with bloating and digestive issues, while also being the primary caregivers and supporters. It dawned on me: this compulsion to "be nice" is yet another trap that is literally killing us.

So here's my invitation to you: For the sake of your health, learn to embrace being a "bitch," if that's what society calls an uncaged woman who breaks free from these chains. If standing up for yourself, setting boundaries, and prioritizing your well-being earns you that label, then so be it. Wear it with pride.

Say no to something minor and build up your confidence so that you can say "no" or "enough" for something much bigger. Because if you don't, your body will, for you. You are powerful, capable, and deserving of respect and self-care. Embracing your true self, with all its strengths and vulnerabilities, is the most authentic form of bravery. Remember, every step you take toward asserting your needs and emotions is a step towards a healthier, more fulfilled you.

You're not alone in this journey—there's a whole community of women walking this path with you. Together, let's redefine strength not as being emotionally available and resilient for everyone else but as honoring ourselves. You've got this!

Heal Stress With Anger

"I never get angry, I just grow a tumor."

—Woody Allen

There is so much judgment against women who get angry in today's society. And I'm not just talking about external judgment; we can also beat *ourselves* up with guilt and shame for "cracking."

What do we tend to do instead? We repress those "unacceptable" emotions—especially anger. And any emotion you repress will express itself as a disease. This could be a subject for a whole new book, but I feel it's important to touch on this topic. I didn't realize how serious my own unresolved anger was until I had consistent stomach issues during an extremely emotionally charged period of my life.

I booked a session with a friend of mine, a holistic practitioner and energy healer called Dr. G, and told him about my stomach issues. Instead of asking what I'd been eating or if I'd had any blood work or food sensitivity tests done, he asked me about my background, my relationship with my parents, when the last time I had cried was, and what my relationship was like with my emotions.

Dr. G offered to help me process my emotions, and I was intrigued. I had recently started training to be a somatic coach ("somatic" means connected to the body). I knew that you can have the most perfect diet, but if you don't process your emotions, they get stored in the body and manifest as disease. Traditional Chinese medicine talks about it a lot, and I was very aware of the correlation—but not of the somatic issues in my own life.

Following Dr. G's instructions, I lay down on the massage table and made the loudest scream I possibly could from deep in my stomach. I did my best, but my voice didn't last longer than 10 to 15 seconds. He touched my belly and asked me to recall anybody who came to my mind. Then he asked me when was the last time I got really pissed at something or somebody.

I told him that I'm not a very angry person. He responded, "Was your dad an angry man?"

Oh.

Yes, in fact, he was.

After an hour and a half of working with Dr. G, he remarked, "I am great at reading people. I can look at someone at a party and tell if they are sad, powerless, or angry without even speaking to them, but with you, it was different. I would never pin you as a person who has deeply repressed anger. You have become very good at hiding it."

Then, all of a sudden, Dr. G made growling noises and shook a pillow in my direction. This sign of anger made me pull back in a panic. He dropped the pillow and returned to his normal tone and posture. "The fact that my anger makes you uncomfortable is because you haven't faced your own."

I raised an eyebrow. He continued: "All you know about anger is the anger your dad directed at other people (yourself or your mom), and it's one of the most misunderstood emotions. Anger is healthy if it's felt in a safe setting. It gets us to do things and ask for more and not settle for mediocre or abusive dynamics. Without anger, no social changes would ever happen."

Dr. G gave me homework to do. I had to start an anger station in my home to have a safe place to be able to get the anger out of my body. It could be any safe means to get the anger out, such as a foam bat to hit into some pillows, a punching bag, or even just a space to take a pillow and scream into it as loudly as possible. I followed his instructions, and do you know what? Releasing healthy anger in the right environment has made me feel much less stressed and overwhelmed. It was a great biohack, and I'd strongly urge you to try it.

Heal Stress With Forgiveness

"Holding a grudge is like drinking poison and waiting for the other person to get sick."

—unknown

When Dave Asprey invited me to do his 40 Years of Zen program, I immediately began searching for flights to Seattle. This had been on my vision board since Dave had been on my podcast, and I couldn't wait. It promises to condense 40 years of meditation into five days and shows a normal (i.e., non-monk) person what zen feels like. "I am so ready for Aggie 2.0," I told him. "I am ready to give less fucks." *Aren't we all?*

The week before, at his advice, I avoided caffeine, social media, work emails—anything that could distract me from being wholly present. By the time I arrived, I was absolutely ready to go. The first thing the coordinator did when she greeted me was to offer me slippers and decaf bulletproof coffee.

The group was super intimate: three people, including myself, plus our coach Heather. We get our brains scanned to know what our baseline is, then prepare to spend most of the week inside a set of futuristic-looking pods with our brains plugged into a massive computer. Each session will take between 90-120 minutes, and we will do multiple sessions daily. Inside the pod was a chair so comfy that it made me sleepy, so I opted to sit on the floor instead, a box of tissues by my side (much-needed, as I found out later); face mist to help keep me alert if I get sleepy; a blanket to help me feel safe and hidden, if need be; and a panic button to call staff if needed. The entire time, our brain was connected to a machine that primes the brain into the alpha state.

There are five main types of brain waves, each associated with different states of consciousness, activities, or moods.

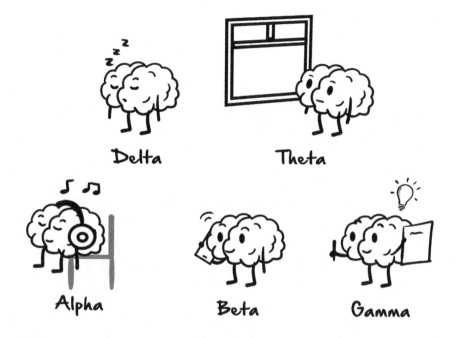

Delta Waves (0.5–4 Hz): These indicate deep, dreamless sleep or unconsciousness.

Theta Waves (4–8 Hz): A bit faster than Delta waves, Theta waves are usually linked with light sleep or daydreaming.

Alpha Waves (8–14 Hz): You'll experience these when you're awake but relaxed, like when you're chilling out with your eyes closed but aren't asleep or meditating.

Beta Waves (14–30 Hz): These are your "doing stuff" brain waves, like during active thinking, problem-solving, and decision-making. Also, being on your phone and after drinking coffee.

Gamma Waves (30–100 Hz): The highest frequency, these trigger perception, problem-solving, and creating mental associations. They're the "Aha!" moment brain waves.

Heather says that our goal for this week is to stay in alpha as much as possible, and then she walks us through the reset process.

Step 1. Call in your guide.
This is usually someone or something you don't know personally. You let them come to you to walk you through this process. For some people, it can be Jesus; for some, it could be a tiger. For me, it was an oak tree.

Step 2. Go to the situation.
Recall a moment from your early life that upset you—that made you either sad, angry, or overwhelmed. Where were you? What were you wearing? What about the other person? What was the temperature of your environment? Recall as many details as possible.

Step 3. State the charge.
Imagine coming up to that person and stating the charge from the place of a wounded five-year-old. Say: *Mom, when you constantly compare my looks to other girls in school, it makes me feel worthless and unlovable;* or *Abuser, when you harmed and threatened me, you made me feel unsafe in my own body.* (From a spiritual perspective, no one can make you feel anything. We allow people to make us think a certain way because we deep down feel that about ourselves, but your inner five-year-old doesn't know that yet, so we will stick with expressions like "You made me feel X, Y and Z.")

Step 4: Feel the feelings.
Allow your wounded inner child to feel anything that comes up. This was the hardest part for me because I had always learned to experience life from the neck up—think about my feelings, analyze them in my head, and try to make sense of them by turning them over in my mind. But feelings happen in the body, too. "Wow, that comment made my chest hurt and tightened my throat." "That incident made my stomach drop and my legs go numb." These were all

sensations I never allowed myself to experience. Letting ourselves feel those without the need to push them away or change them or judge ourselves for it—giving ourselves permission to be "petty" and allowing all the spectrum of emotions was so scary and so freeing.

Step 5: Find the gift.
This is where we were encouraged to *lean into the why and look for something deeper that came out of that childhood moment.* I believe we attract every situation into our life because our soul wants us to feel and grow and direct us toward our true nature. There is always a gift—always a reason—even when we may not see it yet. Something as simple as "It taught me I never want to feel like that again" or "This person being cruel to me made me kinder in the long run" can be a gift as we consider how these painful events shaped us into someone better.

Step 6: Forgive all the way through to love.
Now that we let ourselves feel it all and see the gift of the situation, we allow the spark of forgiveness to slowly soften our hearts.

Step 7: Ask your guide "Are we done yet?"
Before you go, check with your guide to see if it's all resolved. Sometimes the answer is no, and you need to delve a little deeper. That's okay.

The first day or two of this training, I felt like I had no one to forgive. I wondered what I was going to do for the rest of the week, deep in the Washington woods with no phone.

But by Day 3, I broke.

I not only had a lot to forgive others for (even though I was always making up excuses for them instead of holding them accountable), but I also had to forgive myself. And that was the hardest part.

I had to forgive myself for not starting on this healing journey sooner.

I had to forgive myself for not working hard enough and for working too hard.

I had to forgive myself for not always doing my best.

I had to forgive myself for not saying goodbye to my grandpa before he passed away.

The list was endless. I cried and cried, and as I released this bottled-up pain, my brain waves were finally making the move to a more relaxed alpha state. I was getting my 40 years of zen, after all! I was allowing my body to let go of what had kept it tense, worried, and scared for so many years, and it learned how to be present with pain while remaining in an alpha state of calm.

On Friday, I left that training lighter and more in love with myself because I accepted my humanness. As much as I try to do my best, whether with fitness, relationships, or even writing this book, I am only human. And I don't have to forgive myself for that.

Heal Stress With (Self) Love

You know how I said that the hardest part of the 40 Years of Zen training was forgiving myself? Who, exactly, was I forgiving when I looked inside myself?

I was talking about my Perfect Self and my Higher Self. My Perfect Self is the part of me who wants perfection because she thinks perfection will equal love. It comes across as this really mean commanding voice, "Come on Aggie, this should have been perfect."

And then there is my soul self, my Higher Self. When I tap into that higher self, I feel so much more relaxed. I love myself, not despite my mistakes but because of them. Even if my relationships aren't perfect, or my finances might not be where I want them to be, or my followers are disappointed because of what I said or didn't say, I can choose to act from a place of my higher self instead of my perfect self because the perfect self definitely stresses me out.

Perfect Self is the wounded, toxic masculine energy within you (not to be confused with healthy masculine energy). She strives for a perfect body, following an insane meal plan to a T and getting herself to the gym regardless of her exhaustion. She is the mean girl in school, Cruella DeVille, or the general at a Navy SEALs boot camp. She doesn't care how you feel, she only cares about your results. Sure, she's successful in getting the job done, but she makes you resent yourself along the way. She is not willing to forgive you for any mistakes but insists on keeping you hostage.

On the other hand, your Higher Self is your soul, who is waiting for you to start playing big in life and knowing she can't get there without a healthy body. She is also super aware it is her purpose, her mindset, and living to her fullest potential that puts the "cherry on top" in life. That's how you become limitless, my Queen. That's how we change the system. Your Highest Self is generously forgiving but also realizes you never needed to forgive yourself in the first place. She holds a spiritual mindset, as outlined in *Radical Forgiveness* by Colin Tipping. She sees the bigger picture and is filled with compassion and grace.

Heal Stress With Community

In today's fast-paced world, where technology promises connectivity, we often find ourselves more isolated than ever. This growing sense of disconnection (which is paradoxical in an age of hyperconnectivity) has significant implications for our stress levels. The irony of our current era is that while we are constantly in touch digitally, genuine and meaningful connections are becoming rarer.

Social media, rather than bringing us closer, can sometimes deepen our sense of isolation, leading to increased stress and anxiety. The emphasis on individual success and self-reliance in modern culture often overlooks the inherent human need for community and shared experience.

Community plays a critical role in mitigating stress. Being part of a group provides us with a sense of belonging and shared identity, which can significantly reduce feelings of loneliness and isolation. In a community, we find not just social interaction but emotional support, a safe space to express ourselves, and a shared pool of wisdom and coping strategies for dealing with life's challenges. This communal support system is essential for our mental and emotional well-being, helping us to manage and alleviate stress.

I always craved real community and have to say that I am slowly growing into a wonderful group of friends who fill my every day with a lot of joy both in Bali and in LA. Does it require work? Sure, it does. But catching up with your bestie while writing it off as a healing technique is a power move.

Heal Stress With Breathwork

Breathwork? Yup. It's that unglamorous biohack that's as cheap as it gets—but that was my promise to you, that we would talk about hacks that move the needle without you even having to open your wallet. Breathwork is cheap, effective, and (oddly enough) a real game changer. We learned a little about breath earlier, but let's dive in deeper now.

Breathwork earned its spot in my Fit as F*ck Challenge for good reason, but believe me, it didn't win me over right away. When I first connected with Lukis Mac and Hellé Weston, breathwork to me was just tedious. The thought of a two-hour breathing marathon in Venice, CA, sounded like a snorefest, even with these two pros.

Hellè and Lukis are the breathwork masters to the stars; they have worked with Travis Barker, the Kardashians, Megan Fox, and Jake Paul, just to name a few. You might expect them to look like old hippies or some kind of organic nature spirits, but Lukis is covered in tattoos from head to toe and looks like someone you don't want to meet in a dark alley one-on-one. I admit that I was taken aback the first time I met him, yet he's one of the kindest, gentlest, most soulful humans I know. Hellè, now a dear friend of mine, is an angel in human form and truly a badass facilitator.

But my change of heart came later after I got to know them. At first, I was operating under my old assumptions, and when they laid us all side by side on the floor and told us that for the next two hours, we would be breathing only through our mouths as much as possible, I couldn't think of anything more boring. But 20 minutes in, things got real. Weird tingles, hands cramping up like some sort of T-Rex—okay, so this wasn't boring, but it also was not exactly my idea of a chill session.

The next thing I knew, emotions started bubbling up. Hellé was walking around calmly, urging us to keep going. As it turns out, she was onto something—this was more than just breathing. Afterward, Hellè explained, "Every time we have an unprocessed emotion or a stressful event that we don't have the time, energy, or awareness to fully process, we store it in our body as an emotional knot. When we do breathwork, we massage those emotional knots just like a good masseuse can do to loosen up any knots in our back. Many of these unprocessed feelings come up as diseases such as gut issues. The moment I start breathing, I no longer have IBS and indigestion."

Oh. Wow. Well, when you put it that way ...

Most folks dodge breathwork like they do a healthy diet or meditation; it's always a "later" thing. And that's okay; we talked about the power of "yet" back in Chapter 5, remember? I get it; I was reluctant, too, even when *Breath: The New Science of a Lost Art* landed on my radar. "A whole book on breathing? Please." I thought, "How can someone write 300 pages about the most basic human activity? It should be just one sentence: *Hey, you should breathe more. The more oxygen, the better. The end.*"

Well, the book not only ended up being one of my favorites, but when I went to the Beyoncé concert that marked the opening of Atlantis The Royal in Dubai, I actually had the book stashed in my handbag because I couldn't stop reading!

The kicker? Breathing less is key to better health, like ditching the snacking habit but with oxygen. (But you should be thoughtful about taking it in, not choosing to skip it, like with snacks. Definitely don't ditch breathing for better health. That's not how it works. Look, just trust me that developing good breathwork habits is a solid biohack, okay?)

The magic number to aim for is roughly 5.5 breaths a minute. Nose breathing is your chill mode—think about staying grounded and calm and trying for even better posture.

Mouth breathing, on the other hand, is your energy kick—a bit of deliberate stress to train your body to relax on cue. (Remember the hormetic stress discussion?)

And while we're at it, let's talk nostrils—left versus right. It's all about balance, like yin and yang. Left for calm, right for energy, and your body's smart enough to toggle between the two without a manual. No fancy gear is needed; this is just you and your breath, tapping into a mix of relaxation and a mini workout for your lungs.

In short, breathwork isn't just about taking in air—it's about rebooting your system, ditching the stress, and syncing up with life's rhythm.

If you want breathwork for stress, box breathing is a great technique for stress management. This simple exercise involves breathing in slowly through your nose for four seconds, holding your breath for four seconds, gently exhaling through your mouth for four seconds, and then holding your breath again for another four seconds.

Repeating this cycle for a few minutes can significantly calm your mind. It's particularly beneficial for stress relief as it helps regulate the nervous system, shifting you from "fight or flight" mode to a more relaxed "rest and digest" state. This makes it an ideal practice for moments when you need to quickly alleviate stress.

Heal Stress With Meditation

" A true measure of success is a calm nervous system."

–Drew Barrymore

Remember when we talked about fasting? I like to think of meditation as fasting for the soul and mind. It's about taking a moment to stop constantly consuming information and pausing to just be in our feminine energy.

Meditation is an absolute game changer. It's simple, yet its effects are anything but. It's the biohack that doesn't scream for attention, and doesn't demand special gear, yet it rewires your brain, chills out your stress response, and sharpens your focus. It's like lifting weights for your mental health. Seriously, *it's that potent.*

I used to bounce around with meditation, trying this style and that. I got my feet wet with the classics, like transcendental meditation— you know, the type where you get your own secret mantra and repeat it like a magic word? Cool, sure, but it didn't quite fit like a glove for me. Then came Ziva Meditation, courtesy of my friend Emily Fletcher, and that's when everything clicked into place.

I love that Ziva incorporates mindfulness, meditation, *and* manifestation. It resonates with me because I love Emily's philosophy that "We meditate not to get better at meditation; we meditate to get better at *life*."

Explore the various types of meditation out there to find one that works for you. And if you are not in love with meditating, sitting down and giving your mind a break from constantly consuming images, music, and content by simply having your eyes closed can be incredibly helpful and healing.

Heal Stress With Play

I have to admit that I'm still a student when it comes to play. I remember that I loved to play all the time as a child, but somewhere along the way, all the "shoulds" seemed to have gotten in the way. I should be working harder. I should act like an adult. I should be focusing on my work. I should _____ . I'm sure you can fill in the blank. It is part of the brainwashing in our society that it is better to be doing, doing, doing.

The sad truth is when we lose our sense of being able to have fun and play, we harden.

I believe that play is one of the missing pieces for many people. It is absolutely essential for a fulfilling life. If you are reading this book, you are probably an overachiever, multitasking all the time, which is fantastic. Good for you!

But please allow me to ask you a serious question: When was the last time you allowed yourself free rein to play for an entire day—no phone, no emails, no hidden agenda or secretly planning something else in the back of your head—just flat-out play? And now allow me to pose a follow-up: When was the last time you allowed yourself a day like that—*with zero guilt attached*?

I love my work so much, so I used to feel like I didn't need a day off. I would just go, go, go all the time, never pausing to catch my breath or allowing myself a chance to step away for a minute. But this led to extreme burnout that made me worry if I could ever be creative again. Then, I stopped wanting to work at all. I would get self-discipline mixed up with being burned out from trying to do too much all the time. I thought if I was taking time off, I was being lazy.

I never prioritized play. It was something other people did when they didn't know what to do with their lives while *Don't mind me; I'm just over here working away, like a responsible adult.* Then I started listening to Brené Brown and her discussions about the importance of play—and the research behind it. That got my attention! I thought, "I can just do this play thing for 30 minutes, and then I will be more productive. That's what the research says." And that was the approach I tried at first, and it helped—a little. But a 30-minute play break here and there is not enough to fully recharge and revitalize you from all the ways that pushing yourself to do more has depleted you.

Over the years, I have learned how true this saying is, "We don't stop playing because we grow old; we grow old because we stop playing." I started to see that age is just a number and youthfulness comes from our energy. Life is too short to always be serious. I didn't want to be a stressed-out, angry woman anymore. I wanted to be playful, silly, the person who lights up the room with her ability to play. That light is what draws others to us. That feminine energy helps to ground our identity in something other than what we produce.

A common "self-improvement" tip is to listen to a podcast on the way to work rather than listening to music to constantly learn a new skill or expand your knowledge about a given subject. We have become these super productive machines where all of our actions have to make sense. Each move we make has to be attached to creating value. Where literally every second of the day has to be contributing to our growth.

That is literally the opposite of play.

I looked up the definition of play: "Play is an action that brings you a significant amount of joy *without* offering a specific result. It should feel silly, unproductive, and time-consuming."

The best advice I can offer you to spark a sense of play in your life is to start a *to-feel* list that you treat as equally important as your to-do list. Schedule it into your daily routine to help you feel more creative and refreshed.

If you are unsure of where to start, watch kids play; it is second nature for them. Let them teach you how to be a kid again and remind you that you are just a big kid, too.

Get in touch with your inner child. What did you love to do when you were a kid? Listen to that small voice inside you that wants to play—what will fulfill her soul? Take time to make her happy and to fill up her cup. I have a photo of myself at age seven as my phone's wallpaper; this is my reminder that little Aggie is the only person I want to make proud.

As we get older, our ego doesn't want to look silly, especially around others, but our inner child still just wants to be silly and play. If other people laugh at you or are critical of you, remember that they are probably talking to their inner child in that same way, and they deserve our pity. Maybe even aim to gently and kindly embarrass people and make them a little uncomfortable in the hopes of bringing their stifled inner child back.

Heal Stress With Pleasure

A big part of stepping into my power and taking care of my health was reclaiming my pleasure and my pussy. I intentionally didn't "*" the word, nor did I call it "vagina" or "vulva" or anything else. That was an intentional move inspired by the work of Regena Thomashauer (aka, Mama Gena). Her book, *Pussy: A Reclamation,* is one of my favorites because she intentionally uses the word "pussy" because it has historically been used in derogatory or objectifying contexts to shame women, especially in the patriarchal society we live in. Her goal is for us to take back our power by refusing to be shamed by social pressures or sexist ideas. Here we are, proud own-ers of pussies, brave, strong—as well as scared and triggered by the word. Don't feel bad; I am triggered, too, but I am working through it. Wouldn't it be worth challenging the shame and stigma often associated with not only the word but female bodies in general?

Raised in a conservative environment in Poland, pleasure was a taboo topic for me growing up. For too long, I put others' pleasure before mine, following a deep-seated belief that selflessness was the only way to be loved. In my journey of exploring Tantra, I under-stood that I have to claim my power back, and I can't do it without truly claiming my pleasure back. After a professional Yoni massage, I unlocked my sexual "glass ceiling." I now know that orgasms can last hours, and I can get as many as 40 a night. (And if I can, you can too; it just takes a little practice and a lot of breathing!)

Here we are, adult women, scared of and shamed for our own plea-sure, feeling so insecure in bed that we fake orgasms (*yeah, I've been there*), taking the blame on ourselves when we can't climax with a partner. And worst of all, we lay there thinking, "It's okay, I can live without pleasure." But what if we move pleasure from the "Wouldn't it be nice?" category to "It's doctor's orders"?

From a biological standpoint, orgasms reduce stress. Research pub-lished in the *Journal of Biological Psychology* shows that sexual activity can lower blood pressure and reduce stress. The release of oxytocin during orgasm is particularly influential in promoting relaxation and reducing the stress hormone cortisol. Orgasms can also act as a natural pain reliever. A study published in the *Public Library of Science* found that vaginal stimulation significantly increased a woman's pain threshold. This is thought to be due to the release of endorphins during orgasm, which are the body's natural painkillers.

The release of hormones like oxytocin and prolactin following orgasm can promote relaxation and sleepiness. A study in the *Journal of Sleep Research* suggests that sexual activity and orgasm can help improve sleep quality, which we know is crucial for overall health. Regular sexual activity, including orgasm, might also have immune-boosting benefits. A study at Wilkes University found that individuals who had sex once or twice a week had higher levels of immunoglobulin A (IgA), an antibody that helps protect against infections. There's also evidence linking sexual activity and improved mental health. The endorphins released during orgasm can boost mood and create a sense of well-being, potentially helping to reduce symptoms of anxiety and depression.

So if you ever think that your pleasure is secondary or unimportant or negotiable in any way, I want you to remember that it is *literally* part of healthy living. Don't be afraid to ask for (or receive) the pleasure you deserve. Prioritize the pussy!

Heal Stress With Mindset

You know what's stressful? Thinking about all the crap that is happening that threatens to derail your dreams for yourself. I can't begin to tell you how many times the life of *this* book has been sabotaged.

My first reaction? *Why is this happening to me?* Yes, the victim mentality is my knee-jerk reaction, but I am learning how to reframe my thoughts. Things do not just happen "to you" or "to me." They happen *for* us. Remember that you have agency, so believe in your ability to control your life and the events that affect you.

Think about the difference between a sailboat and a raft. (This coming from someone who spent a year sailing across the Pacific from

Mexico to Australia.) A raft is blown around by currents and wind, drifting aimlessly. It has no control over its direction or destination, which is determined by external forces.

In contrast, a sailboat has a sail and a rudder, so it can use the power of the wind and seas to navigate in the direction it wants to go. The person sailing the boat has control over the boat's speed, course, and destination.

You can choose whether you want to be a raft, tossed around by outside circumstances and feeling like a victim, or the sailor of your sailboat, controlling your direction and destiny by navigating toward your desired outcomes, using the circumstances of your life as the things that push your forward.

All of us who set goals have a vision, and part of creating a vision for ourselves is thinking about how we take the internally invisible and make it externally visible. Our mindset is about framing the lens we use to look at the world.

When Things Go Sideways

My alarm goes off as usual around 6 a.m. in LA. As I turn it off, my heart skips as I see a message on my phone—one I will remember forever.

"I have cancer," the message says. Nothing else.

My very best friend has breast cancer. Cancer that came after a long battle with hormones.

How is it fair that one of the nicest people out there, who never complains and never gets angry, is so sick so young?

Whether it's nutrition, emotions, or somewhere in between, I never want to get another message like that one. I never again want to see someone else suffer like that—or to feel my own pain as I suffer alongside them.

I can't make promises about exactly what your health future will look like, but I can encourage you to pursue the healthiest and most beneficial route that I know of. If I can help even one woman resolve her hormone issues, painful periods, or a life of struggling with her body, then I'll keep writing books like this, interviewing experts on my podcast, and posting what I've learned to social media.

All I ask is that you listen to your body and reclaim your power over your health. Take whatever steps you can, whether it's changing the way you eat, trying a new sleep routine, or releasing your pent-up emotional trauma. Just take the first step. Try something new to see if it makes a difference in your overall well-being. Even a minor change can have a massive impact on your long-term health.

Main Character Energy

Close your eyes and imagine your life is a movie. Zoom out a little, and you will see yourself reading this book from above, like a director.

Insert some vibey suspense music in the background, bring up some nice lighting on your face, then zoom back in for a close-up of your eyes suddenly coming alive with the realization that *you are not a background character*.

In fact, not only do you have a speaking role—you are the main character in a film called *My Wonderful Life*! You didn't realize it until now, but it's all good. We're just getting started.

Now, let's make this movie—and your role—Oscar-worthy.

Start bringing main character energy into every single situation of your day-to-day life, because the camera crew is following you everywhere. You're at the store picking your vegetables? At the gym working out? Having a conversation with your boss? Walk with confidence, speak your truth, and act as if you know your worth. (We're getting there.)

The truth is, your freedom, your Higher Self, and your life of abundance all lie on the other side of what makes sense to the world. Their opinions don't matter. The decisions just have to make sense to *your* storyline of a brave, confident, courageous woman who finally went for it.

Think about it: What are the highlights of your life? Falling in love? Going on a solo trip for the first time? Making a huge career move for the sake of your dreams? Aren't they the things that don't really "make sense"? Even if you haven't ever put yourself first and did something ridiculous by society's standards, what about a plot twist? Is this the part of the movie where you step into your power and take responsibility for your life in a way no one else saw coming?

If you see yourself as broken or as a victim where life is happening *to* you and others seem to have it easier, different conditions will continue to manifest in your body. If we become the victors of our life and health while adopting these biohacking principles—well, my dear, we're heading straight for the Kodak Theater to pick up the golden guy.

You are the main character of your life. Bring that main character energy into every situation. And start working on your acceptance speech for all the good things you deserve.

KEY TAKEAWAYS

- **Recognize the Value of "Doing Nothing":** Sometimes the best action is inaction. Like Molly's story demonstrates, incorporating moments of rest and relaxation into your routine can lead to significant improvements in well-being and even weight loss.

- **Acknowledge the Impact of Chronic Stress:** Understand that living in a state of constant stress affects your body and mind. It's not just about recognizing acute stress but also addressing the subtle, ongoing stress that impacts health and happiness.

- **Leverage the Power of Breath and Sighs:** Use breathing techniques, like the physiological sigh, to engage your parasympathetic nervous system and manage stress in real-time.

- **Face and Heal Emotional Traumas:** Addressing deep-seated emotions and traumas, as demonstrated through my own experience with Dr. G, can lead to profound personal healing and stress relief.

- **Harness Community and Social Connections:** Emphasize the importance of genuine connections and community in mitigating feelings of isolation and stress, as seen in my experiences in Bali and LA.

- **Adopt a Positive and Proactive Mindset:** Shift from victimhood to agency, using life's challenges as opportunities for growth and direction, similar to the sailboat analogy.

- **Play, Pleasure, and Sexual Health:** Embrace playfulness and acknowledge the health benefits of sexual pleasure and orgasms, challenging societal stigmas and embracing personal well-being.

- **Main Character Energy and Self-Empowerment:** See yourself as the main character of your life, making decisions that prioritize your growth, health, and happiness.

CHAPTER 10

WHAT NOW?

"The most radical act in a sick society is to heal yourself. Then gently help others heal too."

-unknown

Henry Ford once said, "Whether you think you can, or you think you can't, you're right."

Your mindset determines your outcome, so it is your responsibility to yourself to unravel the lies that you may have been taught about yourself and that you may have even repeated to yourself throughout your life. Entertaining an idea doesn't mean it's true, it just means you're giving it your focus and energy. It is your role, as your own best advocate, to reroute that focus away from those self-limiting beliefs.

I want you to take a moment to reflect on everything we've discussed over the past nine chapters, and think about what mindset shifts are resonating for you right now. From adjustments to the order and timing of your meals to the types of food you prioritize to the ways to work with your cycle to maximizing outcomes to the ways you integrate rest, workouts, and healing of all types—each of these levels requires a change in mindset.

But remember that a change doesn't have to be all-encompassing. Maybe you are just ready to focus on managing sleep and stress at the moment—great! Go for it! Maybe all you feel able to focus on at the moment is getting in tune with your cycle so that you can be ready to implement more changes down the road. Good for you!

My point is simply this: By stepping into a growth mindset rather than remaining in a fixed mindset, you are taking that all-important first step. It's the hardest one to take on this entire journey, and I am *so freaking proud of you* for deciding to do it. From this point on, there is literally no limit to where you can go. Just keep choosing *you* each day.

When I first started Travel in Her Shoes, my travel Instagram account, people called me "motivational" and "inspirational." After all, I was the girl who jumped out of planes, sailed across the Pacific in a tiny sailboat, climbed the tallest peaks in the world, lived with remote tribes in the Amazon jungle and Tanzania, and swam with sharks.

I honestly didn't understand why others didn't do those same things—or whatever adventures they wanted to pursue in their lives. It felt super simple to me to just go for it if you really wanted something. That was until my health issues started.

I went from jumping out of airplanes to being unable to get out of bed in the morning without hitting the snooze button at least three times. Whereas I once was up for anything, now I couldn't get through the day without multiple coffees. Going from the Lower East Side in New York, where I lived at the time, to downtown felt like climbing Kilimanjaro: overwhelming and exhausting. And I didn't feel amazing afterward, either. Nothing felt simple, and I definitely didn't feel like I wanted to "go" for anything but sleep or Netflix.

Why was that the case? Because my body and my biology were out of whack. That's when I realized that no amount of motivation can get someone with an unbalanced biology out of a funk. Balancing your biology will make conquering any of your dreams so much easier—and a life of conquering those dreams is exactly what I want for you.

Look, I know from coaching women that "mindset coaching" is kind of bullshit without looking at someone's biology. You can Tony Robbins yourself all you want, but if you have glucose spikes because of constant carb and sugar consumption, eat food that is making you sick, and don't exercise, you will not see the change. You'll feel inspired and uplifted for a moment, but your state of change won't last.

I believe biohacking is only a means to an end. I don't want it to be your end goal. Figuring out how to maximize your body's thriving doesn't amount to much if you don't go out there and *actually effing thrive*. I would love for your end goal to be stepping into your power and living in your fullest expression. I want to see you give zero fucks about what your friends, followers, or family think of you and your lifestyle. I want to see you live so unapologetically that everything you do, no matter how small, is an act of rebellion against the mainstream brainwashing that is making modern women feel small, stressed, and unsure of their power.

But to do that, you have to focus on your biology, brain, insulin, sex hormones, and diet—even if your natural biology is against you (like mine was).

Before I started biohacking, I had no idea that depression, lack of attention, and distracted focus are a brain problem, not a mindset problem.

When Dr. Amen came on my podcast, *Biohacking Bestie*, he was intrigued about my brain. "Do you have depression, obesity, and addiction in your family?" he asked. "Looking at your genetics alone, you should be curled up on a couch, addicted to substances, massively overweight, and afraid to leave the house." But obviously, that isn't the route I took.

Instead, I am a mindset and motivational coach, have 15 percent body fat, teach women how to stay fit, skydive in my free time, and even though I do psychedelics in the ceremonial setting, I don't drink alcohol or have any substance addictions. My genetics were against me ... but I decided to push back against *them*.

I used biohacking to build a better life for myself. It was never about "becoming a biohacker"; I just wanted to become a better version of myself.

Biohacking isn't an end goal. It's common to over-obsess about biohacks, eliminating more and more "life" from your day and filling it with biohacking. Why? Well, first, because it's exciting; it feels like you're doing something big. Secondly, many of us carry a fear of surrender and a need to control. And thirdly, because too often we feel a need to compete with others.

We biohack to live better and longer; we don't live to biohack.
If a hack is making you miserable, stressed, judgmental of others, or causing you to feel superior to somebody because of what you do that they don't (or vice versa), then it's better for you to take a step back from biohacking for a hot second because it's not making your life—or you—any better.

We're not in the biohacking Olympics. No one gets a prize for "winning biohacking." The point of biohacking is not to create yet another cage to control a woman's behavior or to make another woman feel bad—including the one in the mirror.

Sometimes, in our pursuit of a perfect diet or lifestyle, we end up making our lives worse. If your to-do list is so long with all the habits and all the foods you feel like you have to incorporate that you end up stressed out every day—that's not worth it. The way you eat is not supposed to make you feel miserable. And when something feels good, we often think: "This can't be working then. It is supposed to hurt."

Biohacking ego, just like vegan or fitness ego, is a real thing. Please don't finish this book and then go bio-shame your girlfriends because they are on the pill or got their lips done or eat a donut first thing in the morning.

I would wish for every woman to do fewer biohacks and be happier than to do more and hate her life. The goal is to have more energy to be a better friend and human. That's how we start to heal the world.

"You Popped"

Here's the scene: It's May of 2022, and I am having dinner with my friend Masha when she mentions she works with a woman called Adriana, based in Colombia, who is technically a therapist, but in reality, she's more of a spiritual coach.

I am intrigued. I need to speak to someone because I love my friends, but they know the old me too well to help me navigate all the tsunami changes that have happened inside me this year.

I reach out to Adriana, and she offers me a free introductory session so I can "understand her work."

Immediately, I text her back: "I trust my intuition, and something tells me you're exactly the person I need. Let's go straight into a session."

One week later, when we connect over Zoom, I meet a lady in her early 40s with her head wrapped in a turban. I later find out she's going through cancer treatment.

"What do you expect from our sessions?" she asks.

"I love therapy, and I have been testing different therapists for a year now," I explain. "They all make me feel good about myself and feel seen, but it all comes down to 'Ah, your partner is not paying attention to you. Here are some talking points you can use next time you fight.' I don't need a pat on the back, and I don't want to learn how to fight better. I want to know what my part is in this relationship that is causing conflict. I don't want to break up with Jacob and blame him for not seeing me and my needs and not paying attention, only to repeat the pattern with someone new."

Adriana takes a deep breath and then replies: "It's *you* that isn't seeing yourself. It's *you* who isn't paying attention to your needs. You're projecting. Projecting is getting upset with people for not seeing us, not paying attention to our needs, not listening to what we have to say, not being kind to us, or ignoring what we say—when, in fact, we are doing it to ourselves. You're not listening to your needs. You are ignoring your inner voice and inner child. If this weren't true, you wouldn't get triggered when you feel like Jacob isn't doing these things."

Even as she is speaking these words, I know she's right. I don't pay attention to myself. I don't listen to that voice inside of me. I don't consistently meet my own needs. So why do I expect others to do that for me?

Adriana continues: "In reality, you don't feel seen by yourself. You don't take yourself seriously; why would anyone else do so? You probably didn't feel seen by your parents, and no amount of attention from a partner will ever fill that void. The only person who can make you feel seen is yourself. Now, which part of yourself are you truly not seeing?"

We're five minutes into the session, and I feel like Adriana has already rocked my world. I notice myself getting a little defensive, but this is exactly what I wanted: someone brutally honest who will call me out on my shit.

Now, almost two years later, I wait for my session with Adriana every week. She helps me with my relationship with Jacob and with myself and helps me integrate my ayahuasca sittings.

I've realized that I still don't accept a part of myself that is spiritual. I feel like I don't fit in. The more spiritual I become, the less I fit into the mainstream world, which is what my social media career is all about. Supposedly.

I have done a lot of brave things, but being unapologetically myself is the bravest one of all. It's still on my bucket list. I am still scared of my power and my greatness. Hopefully, one of these days, I'll get there.

***

It's late October in LA, and I'm just back from Poland after dancing on *Polish Dancing with the Stars*. I was invited to this ayahuasca ceremony by my friend Jacek, a contestant on a TV show I hosted the year prior in Marbella, Spain.

After the first session, I can't wait to sit again with the grandmother (as ayahuasca is called by the Quechua people because sometimes she is nurturing and loving, and other times she will knock you down with a hard truth that you wouldn't take from anyone else). It's a weird mix of feeling like Christmas morning and "What is this roller coaster I'm about to jump onto?"

I've decided to do a private session with another shaman in Malibu, and this time, the grandmother sends me a beautiful message: "You don't need another piece of paper to start doing what you're doing. What you're teaching and how you help is beyond anything you can ever learn from somebody else. You also don't need one million people to understand your path. Stop living small in the name of strangers on the internet that you'll never meet."

I know exactly what she's referring to. I have recently started sharing my passion for biohacking, but I keep getting negative comments.

"You better stick to traveling." Translation—Stay small and limit yourself to only one thing. You are not allowed to love many things.

"I wish you went back to the old Aggie." Translation—Don't grow; your growth annoys me because it shows me I am not changing at all.

Those are just a few of the kinds of messages I get these days.

I feel very torn because I miss the old Aggie, too, sometimes. A part of me wishes she was comfortable just traveling and taking beautiful photos. But that's the issue with growth. Once you see things, you can't unsee them. Once you experience the feeling of freedom, you will forever have the reference point of what true freedom really is. Once you leave the cage, you don't ever want to go back in.

"You're like popcorn," Adriana told me that week in our session. "You popped, and you can't become a kernel again. You'll be forever unhappy by living your old Aggie life. You can try to shrink, fit in, lie to yourself that it's okay to compromise on your dreams. But that voice will become louder and louder. In ten years, it's going to be unbearable, and you will probably start to numb yourself just to silence it. Work harder, shop more, watch Netflix, drink, or worst of all, project the unfulfilled dreams onto your children."

It's hard to hear, but I know she's right: I popped. And I can't un-pop.

Weirdly enough, a part of me wishes I was happy living the mainstream life society expects of me—what is expected from all women. It seems so much easier sometimes to stay small, but I also know that I will never respect myself if I hide from the light.

A few weeks later, when I sat down with ayahuasca once more, I was brutally shown all the stories I told myself about staying small. The grandmother starts naming them: "You're too short, too young, not smart enough, and not pretty enough. Your English isn't good enough to be worthy of all that success."

Later, it was about my looks again: "You aren't pretty enough, and then you got too old to do X, Y, and Z. Now you probably think that you're not cool enough or spiritual enough to talk about spirituality or don't have the know-how to be a coach."

I look at my hands and arms, and they look like tree bark. I see myself turning into a tree with roots, planting deep inside Mother Earth. She flashes me with every single person I have met in the last ten years: a taxi driver in Hong Kong, a tour guide in the Philippines who showed me a waterfall, and the family in Brazil who let me stay with them in the jungle. I see their lives and how my posts and stories impacted them and how many people went on life-changing trips because of the locations I shared online.

I don't want to see this. I want to see something deeper, something mysterious, something that will change me.

It must be my ego, I think. *I thought I was here to see my true self. My Higher Self. But my ego is getting in the way.*

But here is the thing about the grandmother. She has an incredible ability to remind you of your power and impact on this planet—and then bring you down to your knees to keep you humble.

"It's not ego," she tells me. *"Your soul wants you to remember your power and your strength.* Your "medicine," what you need right now, is not humility, it's courage. *Forget all the stories society made you believe about yourself. You're here to play big. Acknowledge the impact you already have on this planet—you the immigrant, the ugly, short, too-old*

Aggie, or whatever the story you have about yourself. Because that's all they are—stories."

I come out of that experience with a whole new appreciation for who I am and what, exactly, it is that I am building in this life of mine. The truth is, my biohacking sister, the grandmother's message isn't just for me. You chose to believe those limiting stories to justify not leaping into true abundance, too. But the truth is, it doesn't matter if you had a poor upbringing, have an accent, or your parents aren't still together.

In reality, these things that have made me *me* and made you *you* are the things that have made us absolutely perfect to be leaders. A leader isn't someone who has a perfect life or isn't afraid. It's someone who walks their own path without reacting to others' expectations of them.

You need to become the leader of your life. So do I. Let's keep moving forward together.

If you don't own your power, someone else will.
So go … take up space. Live big. We are just getting started.

What's next?

I'm not going to lie, this book is just the tip of the iceberg when it comes to biohacking. My main focus was to prove to you that you don't need to spend any more money to invest in yourself and your health.

Now, my next question is: Is there anything better than your health to invest money into?

I don't think so. You are your best asset and your best investment.

The better you feel, the less likely you're going to want to pull an all-nighter or get drunk, which may be scary for a few months, but eventually, you will either find new ways of connection or find new friends who reflect your new goals and the new you. And if you can't, please come hang with my community of queens. You are so welcome to join our biweekly calls and biohacking and beyond.

And you'll keep asking: what's next?

Well, you'll enter the world of true personalization. It's not uncommon for biohackers to take up to 80 different supplements a day. Our diets miss the nutrients and vitamins we need to feel our best, and supplements are the quickest and most direct way to make up that deficit.

Supplements are like driving a Bugatti instead of walking somewhere; they make your health journey quicker and help you get away with a not-so-perfect diet of eating out, Uber-eating, or whatnot.

I might be biased as I own a supplement company (Biohacking Bestie), and I am obsessed with creating formulas in conjunction with Shawn Wells, who is (IMHO) the world's best formulator.

Which supplements are best? Well, I would highly encourage you to test your hormones, gut, and DNA to match the perfect diet, tailoring your supplement regime to your individual biochemical needs. Because that's what biohacking is: extreme personalization.

Some of the formulas on the Biohacking Bestie menu included *Drop it Like It's Hot* and *Fit as Fuck* (both for metabolism support), *Not Your Sugar Mama* (glucose support), *Glucose Bestie* (apple cider vinegar in capsules so it doesn't damage your teeth), *All You Can Eat* (digestive enzymes and bitters to help break down gluten, dairy, and fats), and our absolute best seller, *Unbloat Me* (for bloating, duh). We are also launching a skin supplement soon that will help you clear up your skin through the gut (the skin-gut connection is a powerful one!). But my favorite brainchild is *Cycle Bestie*, the most cutting-edge hormone-regulating formula on the market. There is a different formula for each phase of your cycle; our goal is to help you regulate your cycle so reliably that you can use natural contraceptives.

You may want to look into some of the advanced biohacking techniques that are often at the cutting edge of science and personal optimization. You may not be able to spend $2 million a year on different treatments the way some people do, but you might want to explore cryotherapy, hyperbaric oxygen therapy, neurofeedback, infrared saunas, pulsed electromagnetic field therapy (PEMF), photobiomodulation, stem cell therapy, nutrigenomics, and ozone therapy.

And, finally, if you liked hanging out together as much as I did, I would love you to join my community. Fit as F*ck is my 21-day biohacking challenge, where we have videos that dive deeper into everything I have shared with you here.

Just remember, as your bestie, you can always reach out to me on Instagram on @aggie.

KEY TAKEAWAYS

- Your health is your best investment; prioritize it, and the rest will follow.
- Biohacking is about extreme personalization, tailoring your eating choices, techniques, and possibly even supplements to your unique needs.
- Embrace self-acceptance and personal growth, even if it means stepping outside your comfort zone.
- Advanced biohacking offers cutting-edge techniques for those seeking to optimize their well-being.
- Join a supportive community and continue your journey to a healthier, more empowered you.

ACKNOWLEDGMENTS

The problem with publishing a book is that the author gets all the credit while the people who have to put up with her during this time get none. So, here is my attempt to make it up to them with these mere acknowledgments.

First, thank you to my fiancé Jacob. Thank you for missing out on morning snuggles and walks because I woke up at 5:30 a.m. each morning to work on this book. I know I wouldn't be anywhere near as patient as you have been if the roles were reversed. Thank you for reminding me of my strength whenever I doubted myself. Thank you for showing me that being a bio-slacker is so much fun. I love eating delicious food around the world with you.

Thank you to my incredible team, especially to my right and left hands, the incredible Charlotte. You know I wouldn't be here without you. Running a business and writing a book while visiting 30 countries a year wouldn't be possible without your support and flexibility with my insane time zones. Charlotte, thank you for always saying, "You write the book; I'll take care of everything else." Thank you, too, for showing me that it's okay to be kind, but I also shouldn't take any sh*t from people.

Thank you to my parents, Anna and Krzysztof Lal, who have been exactly what I needed to become the person I was meant to become. Kocham was bardzo.

Thank you to my big sister Magda (otherwise known as Kiki). You know everything I do is to impress you. You inspire me with your

25,000+ steps a day, cooking the most delicious food on the planet (should we do a cookbook next?), and being an incredible role model to look up to.

Thank you to my editor, Tiffany, who jumped on the project nine days before the deadline and helped me uncover the message of the book from under many words I so love to use.

Thank you, Lara Hemeryck and your team, for approaching me back in early 2023 and ensuring that everything that lives in my head is backed by science. I love our science chats in Bali.

Thank you to my friends, especially John, for reminding me that "I'm already there."

Thank you to my followers and especially the women in my community. Our biweekly calls remind me of why I do what I do. Nothing inspires me more than seeing you thrive.

Thank you to every woman reading this book and taking action toward her healthier self. This is how we make the world a better place.

Thank you to all the experts whose work inspired this book.

Thank you to my friend Dr. Amy Killen for teaching me the terms "bio-slacker" and "rest and receive." You inspire me massively.

Thank you to Shawn Wells, the best supplement formulator in the world and my business partner, for agreeing to create complex supplement formulas that have never been done before and for believing in my vision. Let's change the world together.

If I have come far, it's only because I am standing on the shoulders of giants. I mention a lot of wisdom from the gurus in the space: Dave Asprey (the optimization), Jessie Inchauspé (glucose),

Dr. Mindy Peltz (fasting), Alyssa Vitti (hormones), Anna Cabeca (female hormones), Jim Kwik (brain and mindset), Dr. Andrew Huberman, Dr. Matthew Walker, Dr. Gabor Maté, Dr. Gabrielle Lyon, and Emily Fletcher, just to name a few. If you want to go down the rabbit hole of biohacking, these are great people to follow. Most of them also teach in my online biohacking course, *Fit as F*ck*, which you are always invited to check out.

REFERENCE LIST

Chapter 1

- Aisha Farhana, *Metabolic Consequences of Weight Reduction*, StatPearls - NCBI Bookshelf, July 10, 2023, https://www.ncbi.nlm.nih.gov/books/NBK572145/.

- Chrysoula Boutari et al., "The Effect of Underweight on Female and Male Reproduction," *Metabolism* 107 (June 1, 2020): 154229, https://doi.org/10.1016/j.metabol.2020.154229.

- Evan D. Rosen and Bruce M. Spiegelman, "What We Talk about When We Talk about Fat," *Cell* 156, no. 1–2 (January 1, 2014): 20–44, https://doi.org/10.1016/j.cell.2013.12.012.

- "Exposures Add up – Survey Results," *Environmental Working Group*, (December 15, 2004), https://www.ewg.org/news-insights/news/2004/12/exposures-add-survey-results#.Wg32G1UrJQJ.

- Frederick William Danby, "Nutrition and Aging Skin: Sugar and Glycation," *Clinics in Dermatology* 28, no. 4 (July 1, 2010): 409–11, https://doi.org/10.1016/j.clindermatol.2010.03.018.

- Lewis G. Halsey, José L. Areta, and Karsten Koehler, "Does Eating Less or Exercising More to Reduce Energy Availability Produce Distinct Metabolic Responses?," *Philosophical Transactions of the Royal Society* B 378, no. 1885 (July 24, 2023), https://doi.org/10.1098/rstb.2022.0217.

- Lorenzo Cohen and Alison Jefferies, "Environmental Exposures and Cancer: Using the Precautionary Principle," *Ecancermedicalscience* 13 (April 16, 2019), https://doi.org/10.3332/ecancer.2019.ed91.

- Melissa Bateson and Gillian Pepper, "Food Insecurity as a Cause of Adiposity: Evolutionary and Mechanistic Hypotheses," *Philosophical Transactions of the Royal Society* B 378, no. 1888 (September 4, 2023), https://doi.org/10.1098/rstb.2022.0228.

- Nuala M. Byrne et al., "Does Metabolic Compensation Explain the Majority of Less-than-Expected Weight Loss in Obese Adults during a Short-Term Severe Diet and Exercise Intervention?," *International Journal of Obesity* 36, no. 11 (July 24, 2012): 1472–78, https://doi.org/10.1038/ijo.2012.109.

- Valentina Vicennati et al., "Stress-Related Development of Obesity and Cortisol in Women," *Obesity* 17, no. 9 (September 1, 2009): 1678–83, https://doi.org/10.1038/oby.2009.76.

- Van Sant, Gus. 1997. *Good Will Hunting*. United States: Miramax.

Chapter 2

- Abdullah Saleh Algoblan, Mohammed A Al-Alfi, and Muhammad Zargham Khan, "Mechanism Linking Diabetes Mellitus and Obesity," *Diabetes, Metabolic Syndrome and Obesity: Targets and Therapy*, December 1, 2014, 587, https://doi.org/10.2147/dmso.s67400.

- Alpana Shukla et al., "Carbohydrate-Last Meal Pattern Lowers Postprandial Glucose and Insulin Excursions in Type 2 Diabetes," *BMJ Open Diabetes Research & Care* 5, no. 1 (September 1, 2017): e000440, https://doi.org/10.1136/bmjdrc-2017-000440.

- Amir Hadi et al., "The Effect of Apple Cider Vinegar on Lipid Profiles and Glycemic Parameters: A Systematic Review and

Meta-Analysis of Randomized Clinical Trials," *BMC Complementary Medicine and Therapies* 21, no. 1 (June 29, 2021), https://doi.org/10.1186/s12906-021-03351-w.

- Andrew Reynolds, Ashley P. Akerman, and Jim Mann, "Dietary Fibre and Whole Grains in Diabetes Management: Systematic Review and Meta-Analyses," *PLOS Medicine* 17, no. 3 (March 6, 2020): e1003053, https://doi.org/10.1371/journal.pmed.1003053.

- Chantal Anifa Amisi, "Markers of Insulin Resistance in Polycystic Ovary Syndrome Women: An Update," *World Journal of Diabetes* 13, no. 3 (March 15, 2022): 129–49, https://doi.org/10.4239/wjd.v13.i3.129.

- Elin Östman et al., "Vinegar Supplementation Lowers Glucose and Insulin Responses and Increases Satiety after a Bread Meal in Healthy Subjects," *European Journal of Clinical Nutrition* 59, no. 9 (June 29, 2005): 983–88, https://doi.org/10.1038/sj.ejcn.1602197.

- Ganpule Anjali, et al., "Snacking Behavior and Association with Metabolic Risk Factors in Adults from North and South India." *Journal of Nutrition*, 153(2), (February 15, 2023), 523–531. https://doi.org/10.1016/j.tjnut.2022.12.032

- Heather Hall et al., "Glucotypes Reveal New Patterns of Glucose Dysregulation," *PLOS* Biology 16, no. 7 (July 24, 2018): e2005143, https://doi.org/10.1371/journal.pbio.2005143.

- Jessie Inchauspe, *Glucose Revolution: The Life-Changing Power of Balancing Your Blood Sugar,*" (S&S/Simon Element, 2022), 304.

- Kara L. Breymeyer et al., "Subjective Mood and Energy Levels of Healthy Weight and Overweight/Obese Healthy Adults on High-and Low-Glycemic Load Experimental Diets," *Appetite* 107 (December 1, 2016): 253–59, https://doi.org/10.1016/j.appet.2016.08.008.

- Keyi Xiao et al., "Effect of a High Protein Diet at Breakfast on Postprandial Glucose Level at Dinner Time in Healthy Adults," *Nutrients* 15, no. 1 (December 24, 2022): 85, https://doi.org/10.3390/nu15010085.

- Kines Kasia, and Tina Krupczak, "Nutritional Interventions For Gastroesophageal Reflux, Irritable Bowel Syndrome, and Hypochlorhydria: a Case Report." *Integrative Medicine* (Encinitas, Calif.) 15,4 (August 1, 2016): 49-53. https://www.ncbi.nlm.nih.gov/pmc/articles/PMC4991651/.

- Louise Clamp et al., "Enhanced Insulin Sensitivity in Successful, Long-Term Weight Loss Maintainers Compared with Matched Controls with No Weight Loss History," *Nutrition & Diabetes* 7, no. 6 (June 19, 2017): e282, https://doi.org/10.1038/nutd.2017.31.

- Marriam Ali et al., "Associations between Timing and Duration of Eating and Glucose Metabolism: A Nationally Representative Study in the U.S.," *Nutrients* 15, no. 3 (February 1, 2023): 729, https://doi.org/10.3390/nu15030729.

- Martin Picard, Robert-Paul Juster, and Bruce S. McEwen, "Mitochondrial Allostatic Load Puts the 'gluc' Back in Glucocorticoids," *Nature Reviews Endocrinology* 10, no. 5 (March 25, 2014): 303–10, https://doi.org/10.1038/nrendo.2014.22.

- Michelle Flynn et al., "Transient Intermittent Hyperglycemia Accelerates Atherosclerosis by Promoting Myelopoiesis," *Circulation Research* 127, no. 7 (September 11, 2020): 877–92, https://doi.org/10.1161/circresaha.120.316653.

- Mirian Ayumi Kurauti et al., "Insulin and Aging," in *Vitamins and Hormones*, 2021, 185–219, https://doi.org/10.1016/bs.vh.2020.12.010.

- Patrick Wyatt et al., "Postprandial Glycaemic Dips Predict Appetite and Energy Intake in Healthy Individuals," *Nature*

Metabolism 3, no. 4 (April 12, 2021): 523–29, https://doi.org/10.1038/s42255-021-00383-x.

- Paula Chandler-Laney et al., "Return of Hunger Following a Relatively High Carbohydrate Breakfast Is Associated with Earlier Recorded Glucose Peak and Nadir," *Appetite* 80 (September 1, 2014): 236–41, https://doi.org/10.1016/j.appet.2014.04.031.

- Roma Pahwa, *Chronic inflammation*. (August 7, 2023). StatPearls - NCBI Bookshelf. https://www.ncbi.nlm.nih.gov/books/NBK493173/

- Saeko Imai et al., "Eating Vegetables First Regardless of Eating Speed Has a Significant Reducing Effect on Postprandial Blood Glucose and Insulin in Young Healthy Women: Randomized Controlled Cross-Over Study," *Nutrients* 15, no. 5 (February 26, 2023): 1174, https://doi.org/10.3390/nu15051174.

- Sagar J. Dholariya., *Biochemistry, Fructose Metabolism*, StatPearls - NCBI Bookshelf, (October 17, 2022), https://www.ncbi.nlm.nih.gov/books/NBK576428/.

- Sofus C. Larsen and Berit Lilienthal Heitmann, "More Frequent Intake of Regular Meals and Less Frequent Snacking Are Weakly Associated with Lower Long-Term Gains in Body Mass Index and Fat Mass in Middle-Aged Men and Women," *Journal of Nutrition* 149, no. 5 (May 1, 2019): 824–30, https://doi.org/10.1093/jn/nxy326.

- Tobias Engeroff, David A. Groneberg, and Jan Wilke, "After Dinner Rest a While, After Supper Walk a Mile? A Systematic Review with Meta-Analysis on the Acute Postprandial Glycemic Response to Exercise Before and After Meal Ingestion in Healthy Subjects and Patients with Impaired Glucose Tolerance," *Sports Medicine* 53, no. 4 (January 30, 2023): 849–69, https://doi.org/10.1007/s40279-022-01808-7.

Chapter 3

- Alda Attinà et al., "Fasting: How to Guide," *Nutrients* 13, no. 5 (May 7, 2021): 1570, https://doi.org/10.3390/nu13051570.

- Anna Baumeister et al., "Short-Term Influence of Caffeine and Medium-Chain Triglycerides on Ketogenesis: A Controlled Double-Blind Intervention Study," *Journal of Nutrition and Metabolism* 2021 (June 15, 2021): 1–9, https://doi.org/10.1155/2021/1861567.

- Bartosz Malinowski et al., "Intermittent Fasting in Cardiovascular Disorders—An Overview," *Nutrients* 11, no. 3 (March 20, 2019): 673, https://doi.org/10.3390/nu11030673.

- Biff F. Palmer and Deborah J. Clegg, "Metabolic Flexibility and Its Impact on Health Outcomes," *Mayo Clinic Proceedings* 97, no. 4 (April 1, 2022): 761–76, https://doi.org/10.1016/j.mayocp.2022.01.012.

- Bo Hye Kim et al., "Effects of Intermittent Fasting on the Circulating Levels and Circadian Rhythms of Hormones," *Endocrinology and Metabolism* 36, no. 4 (August 31, 2021): 745–56, https://doi.org/10.3803/enm.2021.405.

- Corey A. Rynders et al., "Effectiveness of Intermittent Fasting and Time-Restricted Feeding Compared to Continuous Energy Restriction for Weight Loss," *Nutrients* 11, no. 10 (October 14, 2019): 2442, https://doi.org/10.3390/nu11102442.

- Evan D. Rosen and Bruce M. Spiegelman, "What We Talk about When We Talk about Fat," *Cell* 156, no. 1–2 (January 1, 2014): 20–44, https://doi.org/10.1016/j.cell.2013.12.012.

- Joe Alcock, Carlo C. Maley, and C. Athena Aktipis, "Is Eating Behavior Manipulated by the Gastrointestinal Microbiota? Evolutionary Pressures and Potential Mechanisms," *BioEssays* 36, no. 10 (August 8, 2014): 940–49, https://doi.org/10.1002/bies.201400071.

- Kaho Nakamura et al., "Eating Dinner Early Improves 24-h Blood Glucose Levels and Boosts Lipid Metabolism after Breakfast the Next Day: A Randomized Cross-Over Trial," *Nutrients* 13, no. 7 (July 15, 2021): 2424, https://doi.org/10.3390/nu13072424.

- Simin Liu et al., "The Health-Promoting Effects and the Mechanism of Intermittent Fasting," *Journal of Diabetes Research* 2023 (March 3, 2023): 1–15, https://doi.org/10.1155/2023/4038546.

- Stephen D. Anton et al., "Flipping the Metabolic Switch: Understanding and Applying the Health Benefits of Fasting," *Obesity* 26, no. 2 (October 31, 2017): 254–68, https://doi.org/10.1002/oby.22065.

- Xiao Tong Teong et al., "Intermittent Fasting plus Early Time-Restricted Eating versus Calorie Restriction and Standard Care in Adults at Risk of Type 2 Diabetes: A Randomized Controlled Trial," *Nature Medicine* 29, no. 4 (April 1, 2023): 963–72, https://doi.org/10.1038/s41591-023-02287-7.

Chapter 4

- Alpana Shukla et al., "Carbohydrate-Last Meal Pattern Lowers Postprandial Glucose and Insulin Excursions in Type 2 Diabetes," *BMJ Open Diabetes Research & Care* 5, no. 1 (September 1, 2017): e000440, https://doi.org/10.1136/bmjdrc-2017-000440.

- Amir Hadi et al., "The Effect of Apple Cider Vinegar on Lipid Profiles and Glycemic Parameters: A Systematic Review and Meta-Analysis of Randomized Clinical Trials," *BMC Complementary Medicine and Therapies* 21, no. 1 (June 29, 2021), https://doi.org/10.1186/s12906-021-03351-w.

- Andrew Reynolds, Ashley P. Akerman, and Jim Mann, "Dietary Fibre and Whole Grains in Diabetes Management: Systematic Review and Meta-Analyses," *PLOS Medicine* 17, no. 3 (March 6, 2020): e1003053, https://doi.org/10.1371/journal.pmed.1003053.

- Bob Fischer and Andy Lamey, "Field Deaths in Plant Agriculture," *Journal of Agricultural & Environmental Ethics* 31, no. 4 (June 15, 2018): 409–28, https://doi.org/10.1007/s10806-018-9733-8.

- Brian Raymond, "Sustainable Food: A Conversation with Jamie Harvie—Executive Director, Institute for a Sustainable Future," *The Permanente Journal* 14, no. 1 (June 1, 2010): 70–77, https://doi.org/10.7812/tpp/09-092.

- Craig S. Stump et al., "The Metabolic Syndrome: Role of Skeletal Muscle Metabolism," *Annals of Medicine* 38, no. 6 (January 1, 2006): 389–402, https://doi.org/10.1080/07853890600888413.

- Danit R. Shahar et al., "Seasonal Variations in Dietary Intake Affect the Consistency of Dietary Assessment," *European Journal of Epidemiology* 17, no. 2 (January 1, 2001): 129–33, https://doi.org/10.1023/a:1017542928978.

- David A. Cleveland, Allison Carruth, and Daniella Mazaroli, "Operationalizing Local Food: Goals, Actions, and Indicators for Alternative Food Systems," *Agriculture and Human Values* 32, no. 2 (September 30, 2014): 281–97, https://doi.org/10.1007/s10460-014-9556-9.

- DeAnna E. Beasley et al., "The Evolution of Stomach Acidity and Its Relevance to the Human Microbiome," *PLOS ONE* 10, no. 7 (July 29, 2015): e0134116, https://doi.org/10.1371/journal.pone.0134116.

- Elyse S. Powell, Lindsey P. Smith-Taillie, and Barry M. Popkin, "Added Sugars Intake across the Distribution of US Children and Adult Consumers: 1977-2012," *Journal of the Academy of Nutrition and Dietetics* 116, no. 10 (October 1, 2016): 1543-1550.e1, https://doi.org/10.1016/j.jand.2016.06.003.

- Eric S. Orwoll et al., "The Importance of Muscle versus Fat Mass in Sarcopenic Obesity: A Re-Evaluation Using D3-Creatine Muscle Mass versus DXA Lean Mass Measurements," *The Journals of Gerontology* 75, no. 7 (May 21, 2020): 1362–68, https://doi.org/10.1093/gerona/glaa064.

- Gabrielle Lyon, *Forever Strong: A New, Science-Based Strategy for Aging Well*, (New York: First Atria Books, 2023), 389.

- James J. DiNicolantonio and James H. O'Keefe, "Importance of Maintaining a Low Omega–6/Omega–3 Ratio for Reducing Inflammation," *Open Heart* 5, no. 2 (November 1, 2018): e000946, https://doi.org/10.1136/openhrt-2018-000946.

- Jamie Dunaev, Charlotte N. Markey, and Paula M. Brochu, "An Attitude of Gratitude: The Effects of Body-Focused Gratitude on Weight Bias Internalization and Body Image," *Body Image* 25 (June 1, 2018): 9–13, https://doi.org/10.1016/j.bodyim.2018.01.006.

- Jess A Gwin et al., "Muscle Protein Synthesis and Whole-Body Protein Turnover Responses to Ingesting Essential Amino Acids, Intact Protein, and Protein-Containing Mixed Meals with Considerations for Energy Deficit," *Nutrients* 12, no. 8 (August 15, 2020): 2457, https://doi.org/10.3390/nu12082457.

- Joongpyo Shim et al., "The Role of Gut Microbiota in T Cell Immunity and Immune Mediated Disorders," *International Journal of Biological Sciences* 19, no. 4 (January 1, 2023): 1178–91, https://doi.org/10.7150/ijbs.79430.

- Joseph Mercola and Christopher R. D'Adamo, "Linoleic Acid: A Narrative Review of the Effects of Increased Intake in the Standard American Diet and Associations with Chronic Disease," *Nutrients* 15, no. 14 (July 13, 2023): 3129, https://doi.org/10.3390/nu15143129.

- Juan a. Raygoza Garay et al., "Gut Microbiome Composition Is Associated with Future Onset of Crohn's Disease in Healthy First-Degree Relatives," *Gastroenterology* 165, no. 3 (September 1, 2023): 670–81, https://doi.org/10.1053/j.gastro.2023.05.032.

- Karla E. Merz and Debbie C. Thurmond, "Role of Skeletal Muscle in Insulin Resistance and Glucose Uptake," *Comprehensive Physiology*, (July 8, 2020), 785–809, https://doi.org/10.1002/cphy.c190029.

- Kim A. Sjøberg et al., "Exercise Increases Human Skeletal Muscle Insulin Sensitivity via Coordinated Increases in Microvascular Perfusion and Molecular Signaling," *Diabetes* 66, no. 6 (March 14, 2017): 1501–10, https://doi.org/10.2337/db16-1327.

- Laura Maria Wallnoefer, Petra Riefler, and Oliver Meixner, "What Drives the Choice of Local Seasonal Food? Analysis of the Importance of Different Key Motives," *Foods* 10, no. 11 (November 6, 2021): 2715, https://doi.org/10.3390/foods10112715.

- Marica Colella et al., "Microbiota Revolution: How Gut Microbes Regulate Our Lives," *World Journal of Gastroenterology* 29, no. 28 (July 28, 2023): 4368–83, https://doi.org/10.3748/wjg.v29.i28.4368.

- Mehdi Barati, Amirali Ghahremani, and Hasan Namdar Ahmadabad, "Intermittent Fasting: A Promising Dietary Intervention for Autoimmune Diseases," *Autoimmunity Reviews* 22, no. 10 (October 1, 2023): 103408, https://doi.org/10.1016/j.autrev.2023.103408.

- Meijun He et al., "Association between Psychosocial Disorders and Gastroesophageal Reflux Disease: A Systematic Review and Meta-Analysis," *Journal of Neurogastroenterology and Motility* 28, no. 2 (April 30, 2022): 212–21, https://doi.org/10.5056/jnm21044.

- Mieke Van Ende, Stefanie Wijnants, and Patrick Van Dijck, "Sugar Sensing and Signaling in Candida Albicans and Candida Glabrata," *Frontiers in Microbiology* 10 (January 30, 2019), https://doi.org/10.3389/fmicb.2019.00099.

- Monica Esquivel, "Nutrition Benefits and Considerations for Whole Foods Plant-Based Eating Patterns," *American Journal of Lifestyle Medicine* 16, no. 3 (April 22, 2022): 284–90, https://doi.org/10.1177/15598276221075992.

- Pepijn Schreinemachers et al., "Farmer Training in Off-Season Vegetables: Effects on Income and Pesticide Use in Bangladesh," *Food Policy* 61 (May 1, 2016): 132–40, https://doi.org/10.1016/j.foodpol.2016.03.002.

- Peter C. Konturek et al., "Stress and the Gut: Pathophysiology, Clinical Consequences, Diagnostic Approach and Treatment Options," *Journal of Physiology and Pharmacology: Aan Official Journal of the Polish Physiological Society*, 62(6), (December 1, 2011): 591–599.

- Ralf Veit et al., "Health, Pleasure, and Fullness: Changing Mindset Affects Brain Responses and Portion Size Selection in Adults with Overweight and Obesity," *International Journal of Obesity* 44, no. 2 (June 18, 2019): 428–37, https://doi.org/10.1038/s41366-019-0400-6.

- Ralph A. DeFronzo and Devjit Tripathy, "Skeletal Muscle Insulin Resistance Is the Primary Defect in Type 2 Diabetes," *Diabetes Care* 32, no. suppl_2 (November 1, 2009): S157–63, https://doi.org/10.2337/dc09-s302.

- Reetta Satokari, "High Intake of Sugar and the Balance between Pro- and Anti-Inflammatory Gut Bacteria," *Nutrients* 12, no. 5 (May 8, 2020): 1348, https://doi.org/10.3390/nu12051348.

- Rishi Megha, Umer Farooq, Peter P. Lopez. *Stress-Induced Gastritis* (StatPearls, 2023). https://www.ncbi.nlm.nih.gov/books/NBK499926/

- Saeko Imai et al., "Eating Vegetables First Regardless of Eating Speed Has a Significant Reducing Effect on Postprandial Blood Glucose and Insulin in Young Healthy Women: Randomized Controlled Cross-Over Study," *Nutrients* 15, no. 5 (February 26, 2023): 1174, https://doi.org/10.3390/nu15051174.

- Shahla M. Wunderlich et al., "Nutritional Quality of Organic, Conventional, and Seasonally Grown Broccoli Using Vitamin C as a Marker," *International Journal of Food Sciences and Nutrition* 59, no. 1 (January 1, 2008): 34–45, https://doi.org/10.1080/09637480701453637.

- Suci Widhiati et al., "The Role of Gut Microbiome in Inflammatory Skin Disorders: A Systematic Review," *Dermatology Reports*, (December 28, 2021), https://doi.org/10.4081/dr.2022.9188.

- Susan Torres and Caryl Nowson, "Relationship between Stress, Eating Behavior, and Obesity," *Nutrition* 23, no. 11–12 (November 1, 2007): 887–94, https://doi.org/10.1016/j.nut.2007.08.008.

- Susanna Buratti et al., "Influence of Cooking Conditions on Nutritional Properties and Sensory Characteristics Interpreted by E-Senses: Case-Study on Selected Vegetables," *Foods* 9, no. 5 (May 9, 2020): 607, https://doi.org/10.3390/foods9050607.

- Szu-Yu Pu et al., "Effects of Oral Collagen for Skin Anti-Aging: A Systematic Review and Meta-Analysis," *Nutrients* 15, no. 9 (April 26, 2023): 2080, https://doi.org/10.3390/nu15092080.

- Terez Shea-Donohue, Bolin Qin, and Allen Smith, "Parasites, Nutrition, Immune Responses and Biology of Metabolic Tissues," *Parasite Immunology* 39, no. 5 (March 22, 2017), https://doi.org/10.1111/pim.12422.

- Theodoro Pérez-Gerdel et al., "Impact of Intermittent Fasting on the Gut Microbiota: A Systematic Review," *Advanced*

Biology 7, no. 8 (March 22, 2023), https://doi.org/10.1002/adbi.202200337.

- Walter J Crinnion. "Organic Foods Contain Higher Levels of Certain Nutrients, Lower Levels of Pesticides, and May Provide Health Benefits For The Consumer." *Alternative Medicine Review: A Journal Of Clinical Therapeutic* (April, 2010) 15(1), 4–12.

- Wangxin Liu et al., "Influence of Cooking Techniques on Food Quality, Digestibility, and Health Risks Regarding Lipid Oxidation," *Food Research International* 167 (May 1, 2023): 112685, https://doi.org/10.1016/j.foodres.2023.112685.

- Yang Yang et al., "Association between Dietary Fiber and Lower Risk of All-Cause Mortality: A Meta-Analysis of Cohort Studies," *American Journal of Epidemiology* 181, no. 2 (January 5, 2015): 83–91, https://doi.org/10.1093/aje/kwu257.

Chapter 5

- Celme Vieira et al., "Effect of Ricinoleic Acid in Acute and Subchronic Experimental Models of Inflammation," *Mediators of Inflammation* 9, no. 5 (January 1, 2000): 223–28, https://doi.org/10.1080/09629350020025737.

- Christos Pezirkianidis et al., "Adult Friendship and Wellbeing: A Systematic Review with Practical Implications," *Frontiers in Psychology* 14 (January 24, 2023), https://doi.org/10.3389/fpsyg.2023.1059057.

- Elena Cristina Scutarașu and Lucia Carmen Trincă, "Heavy Metals in Foods and Beverages: Global Situation, Health Risks and Reduction Methods," *Foods* 12, no. 18 (September 6, 2023): 3340, https://doi.org/10.3390/foods12183340.

- Eliza Knez, Kornelia Kadac-Czapska, and Małgorzata Grembecka, "Effect of Fermentation on the Nutritional Quality of the Selected Vegetables and Legumes and Their Health Effects," *Life* 13, no. 3 (February 27, 2023): 655, https://doi.org/10.3390/life13030655.

- Elizabeth N. Madva et al., "Positive Psychological Well-being: A Novel Concept for Improving Symptoms, Quality of Life, and Health Behaviors in Irritable Bowel Syndrome," *Neurogastroenterology and Motility* 35, no. 4 (January 17, 2023), https://doi.org/10.1111/nmo.14531.

- "Exposures Add up – Survey Results," *Environmental Working Group*, (December 15, 2004), https://www.ewg.org/news-insights/news/2004/12/exposures-add-survey-results#.Wg32G1UrJQJ.

- Farhad Vahid et al., "Pro- and Antioxidant Effect of Food Items and Matrices during Simulated In Vitro Digestion," *Foods* 12, no. 8 (April 20, 2023): 1719, https://doi.org/10.3390/foods12081719.

- Fatima S. Poswal et al., "Herbal Teas and Their Health Benefits: A Scoping Review," *Plant Foods for Human Nutrition* 74, no. 3 (June 26, 2019): 266–76, https://doi.org/10.1007/s11130-019-00750-w.

- Jacqueline A. Barnett and Deanna L. Gibson, "Separating the Empirical Wheat from the Pseudoscientific Chaff: A Critical Review of the Literature Surrounding Glyphosate, Dysbiosis and Wheat-Sensitivity," *Frontiers in Microbiology* 11 (September 25, 2020), https://doi.org/10.3389/fmicb.2020.556729.

- Justine M. Cruz and Jacolin A. Murray, "Determination of Glyphosate and AMPA in Oat Products for the Selection of Candidate Reference Materials," *Food Chemistry* 342 (April 1, 2021): 128213, https://doi.org/10.1016/j.foodchem.2020.128213.

- Karen D. Bradham et al., "A National Survey of Lead and Other Metal(Loids) in Residential Drinking Water in the

United States," *Journal of Exposure Science and Environmental Epidemiology* 33, no. 2 (August 19, 2022): 160–67, https://doi.org/10.1038/s41370-022-00461-6.

- Ksenija Nešić, Kristina Habschied, and Krešimir Mastanjević, "Modified Mycotoxins and Multitoxin Contamination of Food and Feed as Major Analytical Challenges," *Toxins* 15, no. 8 (August 19, 2023): 511, https://doi.org/10.3390/toxins15080511.

- Lorenzo Cohen and Alison Jefferies, "Environmental Exposures and Cancer: Using the Precautionary Principle," *Ecancermedicalscience* 13 (April 16, 2019), https://doi.org/10.3332/ecancer.2019.ed91.

- Marí Van De Vyver, "Immunology of Chronic Low-Grade Inflammation: Relationship with Metabolic Function," *Journal of Endocrinology* 257, no. 1 (January 23, 2023), https://doi.org/10.1530/joe-22-0271.

- Martina Rahe and Petra Jansen, "A Closer Look at the Relationships between Aspects of Connectedness and Flourishing," *Frontiers in Psychology* 14 (March 30, 2023), https://doi.org/10.3389/fpsyg.2023.1137752.

- Nguyen Phan Khoi Le, Markus Jörg Altenburger, and Evelyn Lamy, "Development of an Inflammation-Triggered In Vitro 'Leaky Gut' Model Using Caco-2/HT29-MTX-E12 Combined with Macrophage-like THP-1 Cells or Primary Human-Derived Macrophages," *International Journal of Molecular Sciences* 24, no. 8 (April 18, 2023): 7427, https://doi.org/10.3390/ijms24087427.

- Peter Lehman et al., "Low-Dose Glyphosate Exposure Alters Gut Microbiota Composition and Modulates Gut Homeostasis," *Environmental Toxicology and Pharmacology* 100 (June 1, 2023): 104149, https://doi.org/10.1016/j.etap.2023.104149.

- Philippe Grandjean et al., "Weight Loss Relapse Associated with Exposure to Perfluorinated Alkylate Substances," *Obesity* 31, no. 6 (April 17, 2023): 1686–96, https://doi.org/10.1002/oby.23755.

- Quynh Do et al., "Differential Contributions of Distinct Free Radical Peroxidation Mechanisms to the Induction of Ferroptosis," *JACS Au* 3, no. 4 (March 4, 2023): 1100–1117, https://doi.org/10.1021/jacsau.2c00681.

- Rehana Salim et al., "A Review on Anti-Nutritional Factors: Unraveling the Natural Gateways to Human Health," *Frontiers in Nutrition* 10 (August 31, 2023), https://doi.org/10.3389/fnut.2023.1215873.

- Sachiko Komagata, "Kanpumasatsu: A Superficial Self-Massage with a Dry Towel to Enhance Relaxation and Immune Functions," *Journal of Interprofessional Education and Practice* 31 (June 1, 2023): 100609, https://doi.org/10.1016/j.xjep.2023.100609.

- Solomon Abera, Weldegebriel Yohannes, and Bhagwan Singh Chandravanshi, "Effect of Processing Methods on Antinutritional Factors (Oxalate, Phytate, and Tannin) and Their Interaction with Minerals (Calcium, Iron, and Zinc) in Red, White, and Black Kidney Beans," *International Journal of Analytical Chemistry* (October 18, 2023): 1–11, https://doi.org/10.1155/2023/6762027.

- Süleyman Sezai Yıldız, Ayfer Gözü Pirinçcioğlu, and Enes Arıca, "Evaluation of Heavy Metal (Lead, Mercury, Cadmium, and Manganese) Levels in Blood, Plasma, and Urine of Adolescents with Aggressive Behavior," *Cureus*, (January 17, 2023), https://doi.org/10.7759/cureus.33902.

- Tzu-Rong Peng et al., "Effectiveness of Oil Pulling for Improving Oral Health: A Meta-Analysis," *Healthcare* 10, no. 10 (October 11, 2022): 1991, https://doi.org/10.3390/healthcare10101991.

- Wen-Hui Kuan, Yi-Lang Chen, and Chao-Lin Liu, "Excretion of Ni, Pb, Cu, As, and Hg in Sweat under Two Sweating Conditions," *International Journal of Environmental Research and Public Health* 19, no. 7 (April 4, 2022): 4323, https://doi.org/10.3390/ijerph19074323.
- Yücel Büyükdere and Aslı Akyol, "From a Toxin to an Obesogen: A Review of Potential Obesogenic Roles of Acrylamide with a Mechanistic Approach," *Nutrition Reviews*, (May 8, 2023), https://doi.org/10.1093/nutrit/nuad041.

Chapter 6

- Aqeed Abid Ali and Faruk Hasan Faraj, "Clinicopathological Profile of Mastalgia in Females: Incidence, Types, and Pathological Correlations. a Cross-Sectional Study," *Annals of Medicine and Surgery* 85, no. 10 (August 17, 2023): 4764–72, https://doi.org/10.1097/ms9.0000000000001159.
- Abdurrahman Coşkun, Atefeh Zarepour, and Ali Zarrabi, "Physiological Rhythms and Biological Variation of Biomolecules: The Road to Personalized Laboratory Medicine," *International Journal of Molecular Sciences* 24, no. 7 (March 27, 2023): 6275, https://doi.org/10.3390/ijms24076275.
- Abrams, J.J. Star Wars. (May 25, 1977)
- Alisa Vitti, *In the FLO: Unlock Your Hormonal Advantage and Revolutionize Your Life*, (HarperOne, 2020), 382
- Andressa Gonsioroski, Vasiliki E. Mourikes, and Jodi A. Flaws, "Endocrine Disruptors in Water and Their Effects on the Reproductive System," *International Journal of Molecular Sciences* 21, no. 6 (March 12, 2020): 1929, https://doi.org/10.3390/ijms21061929.

- Angela Lanfranchi, "A Scientific Basis for Humanae Vitae and Natural Law," *The Linacre Quarterly* 85, no. 2 (April 12, 2018): 148–54, https://doi.org/10.1177/0024363918756191.

- Anna Cabeca, *The Hormone Fix: Burn Fat Naturally, Boost Energy, Sleep Better, and Stop Hot Flashes, the Keto-Green Way,* (Ballantine Books, 2019), 400.

- Annika Haufe and Brigitte Leeners, "Sleep Disturbances across a Woman's Lifespan: What Is the Role of Reproductive Hormones?," *Journal of the Endocrine Society* 7, no. 5 (March 6, 2023), https://doi.org/10.1210/jendso/bvad036.

- Benjamin J. Delgado, Wilfredo Lopez-Ojeda,. *Estrogen,* In Stat-Pearls. StatPearls Publishing. (June 26, 2023).

- Beverly G Reed, *The Normal Menstrual Cycle and the Control of Ovulation,* Endotext - NCBI Bookshelf, (August 5, 2018), https://www.ncbi.nlm.nih.gov/books/NBK279054/.

- Brené Brown, *The Gifts of Imperfection: Let Go of Who You Think You're Supposed to Be and Embrace Who You Are,* (Hazelden Publishing, 2010), 188.

- Carolyn M. Matthews, "Nurturing Your Divine Feminine," *Baylor University Medical Center Proceedings* 24, no. 3 (July 1, 2011): 248, https://doi.org/10.1080/08998280.2011.11928725.

- Charlotte Helfrich-Förster et al., "Women Temporarily Synchronize Their Menstrual Cycles with the Luminance and Gravimetric Cycles of the Moon," *Science Advances* 7, no. 5 (January 29, 2021), https://doi.org/10.1126/sciadv.abe1358.

- Dalberg Advisors, Wijnand de Wit and Nathan Bigaud, "No Plastic in Nature: Assessing Plastic Ingestion From Nature to People." (2019). https://d2ouvy59p0dg6k.cloudfront.net/downloads/plastic_ingestion_web_spreads.pdf

- Danielle B. Cooper, Preeti Patel, Heba Mahdy, Oral Contraceptive Pills, In StatPearls. StatPearls Publishing, (November 24, 2022), https://www.ncbi.nlm.nih.gov/books/NBK430882/.

- Dhanalakshmi K. Thiyagarajan, *Physiology, Menstrual Cycle*, StatPearls - NCBI Bookshelf, (October 24, 2022), https://www.ncbi.nlm.nih.gov/books/NBK500020/.

- Divya Kanchibhotla, Saumya Subramanian, and Deeksha Singh, "Management of Dysmenorrhea through Yoga: A Narrative Review," Frontiers in Pain Research 4 (March 30, 2023), https://doi.org/10.3389/fpain.2023.1107669.

- "Documentary Filmmakers | The Business Of Birth Control," Abby Epstein, *The Business Of*, https://www.thebusinessof.life/.

- Etsuro Ito, Rei Shima, and Tohru Yoshioka, "A Novel Role of Oxytocin: Oxytocin-Induced Well-Being in Humans," *Biophysics and Physicobiology* 16, no. 0 (January 1, 2019): 132–39, https://doi.org/10.2142/biophysico.16.0_132.

- Gandhi Rádis-Baptista, "Do Synthetic Fragrances in Personal Care and Household Products Impact Indoor Air Quality and Pose Health Risks?," *Journal of Xenobiotics* 13, no. 1 (March 1, 2023): 121–31, https://doi.org/10.3390/jox13010010.

- Guy W. Fincham et al., "Effect of Breathwork on Stress and Mental Health: A Meta-Analysis of Randomised-Controlled Trials," *Scientific Reports* 13, no. 1 (January 9, 2023), https://doi.org/10.1038/s41598-022-27247-y.

- Hannah Bronfman, "Hormones 101 with Alisa Vitti of Flo Living | HBFIT Wellness," (June 29, 2017), https://www.youtube.com/watch?v=Uw5tVc5WHjc.

- Haolin Zhang et al., "Relationship between Body Composition, Insulin Resistance, and Hormonal Profiles in Women with Polycystic Ovary Syndrome," *Frontiers in Endocrinology* 13 (January 9, 2023), https://doi.org/10.3389/fendo.2022.1085656.

- Hui Yan et al., "Estrogen Improves Insulin Sensitivity and Suppresses Gluconeogenesis via the Transcription Factor Foxo1," *Diabetes* 68, no. 2 (November 27, 2018): 291–304, https://doi.org/10.2337/db18-0638.

- Hui Zhang and Sairam, "Sex Hormone Imbalances and Adipose Tissue Dysfunction Impacting on Metabolic Syndrome; a Paradigm for the Discovery of Novel Adipokines," *Hormone Molecular Biology and Clinical Investigation* 17, no. 2 (February 1, 2014): 89–97, https://doi.org/10.1515/hmbci-2014-0002.

- Junyoung Jo and Sun Haeng Lee, "Heat Therapy for Primary Dysmenorrhea: A Systematic Review and Meta-Analysis of Its Effects on Pain Relief and Quality of Life," *Scientific Reports* 8, no. 1 (November 2, 2018), https://doi.org/10.1038/s41598-018-34303-z.

- Katherine A. Liu and Natalie A. DiPietro Mager, "Women's Involvement in Clinical Trials: Historical Perspective and Future Implications," *Pharmacy Practice*, 14, no. 1 (March 6, 2016): 708, https://doi.org/10.18549/pharmpract.2016.01.708.

- Kathleen C. Light, Karen Grewen, and Janet A. Amico, "More Frequent Partner Hugs and Higher Oxytocin Levels Are Linked to Lower Blood Pressure and Heart Rate in Premenopausal Women," *Biological Psychology* 69, no. 1 (April 1, 2005): 5–21, https://doi.org/10.1016/j.biopsycho.2004.11.002.

- Keiji Inoue and Hiroshi Mikami, "Effects of Simplified Lymph Drainage on the Body: In Females with Menopausal Disorder," *Journal of Physical Therapy Science* 29, no. 1 (January 1, 2017): 115–18, https://doi.org/10.1589/jpts.29.115.

- Lee, Jennifer and Buck, Chris. *Frozen.* (November 19, 2013). Disney Publishing Worldwide.

- Luis Enrique Soria-Jasso et al., "Beneficial and Deleterious Effects of Female Sex Hormones, Oral Contraceptives, and Phytoestrogens by Immunomodulation on the Liver," *International Journal of Molecular Sciences* 20, no. 19 (September 22, 2019): 4694, https://doi.org/10.3390/ijms20194694.

- Małgorzata Stefaniak et al., "Progesterone and Its Metabolites Play a Beneficial Role in Affect Regulation in the Female Brain," *Pharmaceuticals* 16, no. 4 (March 31, 2023): 520, https://doi.org/10.3390/ph16040520.

- Małgorzata Stefaniak et al., "Progesterone and Its Metabolites Play a Beneficial Role in Affect Regulation in the Female Brain," *Pharmaceuticals* 16, no. 4 (March 31, 2023): 520, https://doi.org/10.3390/ph16040520.

- Manuel E. Cortés and Arístides Alfaro, "The Effects of Hormonal Contraceptives on Glycemic Regulation," *The Linacre Quarterly* 81, no. 3 (August 1, 2014): 209–18, https://doi.org/10.1179/2050854914y.0000000023.

- Marija Kundaković and Devin Rocks, "Sex Hormone Fluctuation and Increased Female Risk for Depression and Anxiety Disorders: From Clinical Evidence to Molecular Mechanisms," *Frontiers in Neuroendocrinology* 66 (July 1, 2022): 101010, https://doi.org/10.1016/j.yfrne.2022.101010.

- Markus Heinrichs et al., "Social Support and Oxytocin Interact to Suppress Cortisol and Subjective Responses to Psychosocial Stress," *Biological Psychiatry* 54, no. 12 (December 1, 2003): 1389–98, https://doi.org/10.1016/s0006-3223(03)00465-7.

- Mauri José Piazza and Almir Antônio Urbanetz, "Environmental Toxins and the Impact of Other Endocrine Disrupting Chemicals in Women's Reproductive Health," *JBRA Assisted Reproduction*, (January 1, 2019), https://doi.org/10.5935/1518-0557.20190016.

- Megan Palmery, "Oral Contraceptives and Changes in Nutritional Requirements," *European Review for Medical and Pharmacological Sciences* vol. 17,13 (July 1, 2013): 1804-13.

- Michaela M Rogan and Katherine Black, "Dietary Energy Intake across the Menstrual Cycle: A Narrative Review,"

Nutrition Reviews 81, no. 7 (November 11, 2022): 869–86, https://doi.org/10.1093/nutrit/nuac094.

- Miguel Bellosta-Batalla et al., "Brief Mindfulness Session Improves Mood and Increases Salivary Oxytocin in Psychology Students," *Stress and Health* 36, no. 4 (April 2, 2020): 469–77, https://doi.org/10.1002/smi.2942.

- Miles Campbell, Ishwarlal Jialal, *Physiology, Endocrine Hormones*, In StatPearls. StatPearls Publishing. (September 26, 2022).

- Monica De Paoli, Alexander Zakharia, and Geoff H. Werstuck, "The Role of Estrogen in Insulin Resistance," *American Journal of Pathology* 191, no. 9 (September 1, 2021): 1490–98, https://doi.org/10.1016/j.ajpath.2021.05.011.

- Namyoung Yang and Sang-Dol Kim, "Effects of a Yoga Program on Menstrual Cramps and Menstrual Distress in Undergraduate Students with Primary Dysmenorrhea: A Single-Blind, Randomized Controlled Trial," *Journal of Alternative and Complementary Medicine* 22, no. 9 (September 1, 2016): 732–38, https://doi.org/10.1089/acm.2016.0058.

- Nan Lin et al., "Volatile Organic Compounds in Feminine Hygiene Products Sold in the US Market: A Survey of Products and Health Risks," *Environment International* 144 (November 1, 2020): 105740, https://doi.org/10.1016/j.envint.2020.105740.

- Paola Valbonesi et al., "Contaminants of Emerging Concern in Drinking Water: Quality Assessment by Combining Chemical and Biological Analysis," *Science of the Total Environment* 758 (March 1, 2021): 143624, https://doi.org/10.1016/j.scitotenv.2020.143624.

- Patrick Levallois et al., "Public Health Consequences of Lead in Drinking Water," *Current Environmental Health Reports* 5, no. 2 (March 19, 2018): 255–62, https://doi.org/10.1007/s40572-018-0193-0.

- Paula Recacha-Ponce et al., "Is It Necessary to Adapt Training According to the Menstrual Cycle? Influence of Contraception and Physical Fitness Variables," *Life* 13, no. 8 (August 17, 2023): 1764, https://doi.org/10.3390/life13081764.

- Risa Mitsuhashi et al., "Factors Associated with the Prevalence and Severity of Menstrual-Related Symptoms: A Systematic Review and Meta-Analysis," *International Journal of Environmental Research and Public Health* 20, no. 1 (December 29, 2022): 569, https://doi.org/10.3390/ijerph20010569.

- Rishi Hasan et al., "Effects of Hormones and Endocrine Disorders on Hair Growth," *Cureus*, (December 20, 2022), https://doi.org/10.7759/cureus.32726.

- Rui Zhang et al., "The Relevant of Sex Hormone Levels and Acne Grades in Patients with Acne Vulgaris: A Cross-Sectional Study in Beijing," *Clinical, Cosmetic and Investigational Dermatology* 15 (October 1, 2022): 2211–19, https://doi.org/10.2147/ccid.s385376.

- Sameer Zope and Rakesh A Zope, "Sudarshan Kriya Yoga: Breathing for Health," *International Journal of Yoga* 6, no. 1 (January 1, 2013): 4, https://doi.org/10.4103/0973-6131.105935.

- Sarah K. Rogers et al., "Efficacy of Psychological Interventions for Dysmenorrhea: A Meta-Analysis," *Pain Medicine* 24, no. 9 (May 8, 2023): 1086–99, https://doi.org/10.1093/pm/pnad058.

- Shalini Gainder and Bharti Sharma, "Update on Management of Polycystic Ovarian Syndrome for Dermatologists," *Indian Dermatology Online Journal* 10, no. 2 (January 1, 2019): 97, https://doi.org/10.4103/idoj.idoj_249_17.

- Sorin Tunaru et al., "Castor Oil Induces Laxation and Uterus Contraction via Ricinoleic Acid Activating Prostaglandin EP 3 Receptors," *Proceedings of the National Academy of Sciences of the United States of America* 109, no. 23 (May 21, 2012): 9179–84, https://doi.org/10.1073/pnas.1201627109.

- Stefano Ciardullo et al., "Differential Association of Sex Hormones with Metabolic Parameters and Body Composition in Men and Women from the United States," *Journal of Clinical Medicine* 12, no. 14 (July 19, 2023): 4783, https://doi.org/10.3390/jcm12144783.

- Tinkara Srnovršnik, Irma Virant-Klun, and Bojana Pinter, "Polycystic Ovary Syndrome and Endocrine Disruptors (Bisphenols, Parabens, and Triclosan) — A Systematic Review," *Life* 13, no. 1 (January 4, 2023): 138, https://doi.org/10.3390/life13010138.

- "The FDA Approves the Pill," American Experience, https://www.pbs.org/wgbh/americanexperience/features/pill-us-food-and-drug-administration-approves-pill

Chapter 7

- Aditya Mahindru, Pradeep M. Patil, and Varun Agrawal, "Role of Physical Activity on Mental Health and Well-Being: A Review," *Cureus*, 15 (January 7, 2023): e33475, https://doi.org/10.7759/cureus.33475.

- Aggie Lal, "Cycle Bestie," https://www.cyclebestie.com/cycle-bestie-waitlist.

- Alessio Bellini et al., "Walking Attenuates Postprandial Glycemic Response: What Else Can We Do without Leaving Home or the Office?," *International Journal of Environmental Research and Public Health* 20, no. 1 (December 24, 2022): 253, https://doi.org/10.3390/ijerph20010253.

- Alexandra Vieira et al., "Effects of Aerobic Exercise Performed in Fasted v. Fed State on Fat and Carbohydrate Metabolism in Adults: A Systematic Review and Meta-Analysis," *British Journal of Nutrition* 116, no. 7 (September 9, 2016): 1153–64, https://doi.org/10.1017/s0007114516003160.

- Alia J. Crum and Ellen J. Langer, "Mind-Set Matters," *Psychological Science* 18, no. 2 (February 1, 2007): 165–71, https://doi.org/10.1111/j.1467-9280.2007.01867.x.

- Andrea T. Duran et al., "Breaking Up Prolonged Sitting to Improve Cardiometabolic Risk: Dose–Response Analysis of a Randomized Crossover Trial," *Medicine and Science in Sports and Exercise* 55, no. 5 (January 12, 2023): 847–55, https://doi.org/10.1249/mss.0000000000003109.

- Arnold G. Nelson, Joke Kokkonen, and David A. Arnall, "Twenty Minutes of Passive Stretching Lowers Glucose Levels in an At-Risk Population: An Experimental Study," *Journal of Physiotherapy* 57, no. 3 (January 1, 2011): 173–78, https://doi.org/10.1016/s1836-9553(11)70038-8.

- Cihat Uçar, Tuba Özgöçer, and Sedat Yıldız, "Late-Night Exercise Affects the Autonomic Nervous System Activity but Not the Hypothalamo-Pituitary-Adrenal Axis in the Next Morning," *Journal of Sports Medicine and Physical Fitness* 58, no. 1–2 (November 1, 2017), https://doi.org/10.23736/s0022-4707.16.06766-9.

- Debra L Blackwell, and Tainya C Clarke. "State Variation in Meeting the 2008 Federal Guidelines for Both Aerobic and Muscle-Strengthening Activities through Leisure-Time Physical Activity among Adults Aged 18-64: United States, 2010-2015," *National Health Statistics Reports* (June 1, 2018.): 1-22.

- "Erasing Fears & Traumas Based on the Modern Neuroscience of Fear - Huberman Lab," September 23, 2023, https://www.hubermanlab.com/episode/erasing-fears-and-traumas-based-on-the-modern-neuroscience-of-fear.

- Eric S. Orwoll et al., "The Importance of Muscle versus Fat Mass in Sarcopenic Obesity: A Re-Evaluation Using D3-Creatine Muscle Mass versus DXA Lean Mass Measurements,"

The Journals of Gerontology 75, no. 7 (May 21, 2020): 1362–68, https://doi.org/10.1093/gerona/glaa064.

- Haifeng Zhang et al., "Comparable Effects of High-Intensity Interval Training and Prolonged Continuous Exercise Training on Abdominal Visceral Fat Reduction in Obese Young Women," *Journal of Diabetes Research* 2017 (January 1, 2017): 1–9, https://doi.org/10.1155/2017/5071740.

- I-Min Lee et al., "Association of Step Volume and Intensity with All-Cause Mortality in Older Women," *JAMA Internal Medicine* 179, no. 8 (August 1, 2019): 1105, https://doi.org/10.1001/jamainternmed.2019.0899.

- Julia C. Basso and Wendy Suzuki, "The Effects of Acute Exercise on Mood, Cognition, Neurophysiology, and Neurochemical Pathways: A Review," *Brain Plasticity* 2, no. 2 (March 28, 2017): 127–52, https://doi.org/10.3233/bpl-160040.

- Kaoutar Ennour-Idrissi, Elizabeth Maunsell, and Caroline Diorio, "Effect of Physical Activity on Sex Hormones in Women: A Systematic Review and Meta-Analysis of Randomized Controlled Trials," *Breast Cancer Research* 17, no. 1 (November 5, 2015), https://doi.org/10.1186/s13058-015-0647-3.

- Kim A. Sjøberg et al., "Exercise Increases Human Skeletal Muscle Insulin Sensitivity via Coordinated Increases in Microvascular Perfusion and Molecular Signaling," *Diabetes* 66, no. 6 (March 14, 2017): 1501–10, https://doi.org/10.2337/db16-1327.

- Len De Nys et al., "The Effects of Physical Activity on Cortisol and Sleep: A Systematic Review and Meta-Analysis," *Psychoneuroendocrinology* 143 (September 1, 2022): 105843, https://doi.org/10.1016/j.psyneuen.2022.105843.

- Mark Evans, Karl E. Cogan, and Brendan Egan, "Metabolism of Ketone Bodies during Exercise and Training: Physiological Basis for Exogenous Supplementation," *The Journal of*

Physiology 595, no. 9 (December 7, 2016): 2857–71, https://doi. org/10.1113/jp273185.

- Namyoung Yang and Sang-Dol Kim, "Effects of a Yoga Program on Menstrual Cramps and Menstrual Distress in Undergraduate Students with Primary Dysmenorrhea: A Single-Blind, Randomized Controlled Trial," *Journal of Alternative and Complementary Medicine* 22, no. 9 (September 1, 2016): 732–38, https://doi.org/10.1089/acm.2016.0058.

- Richard S. Metcalfe et al., "Extremely Short Duration Interval Exercise Improves 24-h Glycaemia in Men with Type 2 Diabetes," *European Journal of Applied Physiology* 118, no. 12 (August 31, 2018): 2551–62, https://doi.org/10.1007/s00421-018-3980-2.

- Richard S. Metcalfe et al., "Towards the Minimal Amount of Exercise for Improving Metabolic Health: Beneficial Effects of Reduced-Exertion High-Intensity Interval Training," *European Journal of Applied Physiology* 112, no. 7 (November 29, 2011): 2767–75, https://doi.org/10.1007/s00421-011-2254-z.

- Stephen J. Genuis et al., "Blood, Urine, and Sweat (BUS) Study: Monitoring and Elimination of Bioaccumulated Toxic Elements," *Archives of Environmental Contamination and Toxicology* 61, no. 2 (November 6, 2010): 344–57, https://doi.org/10.1007/s00244-010-9611-5.

- Tanja Oosthuyse and Andrew Bosch, "The Effect of the Menstrual Cycle on Exercise Metabolism," *Sports Medicine* 40, no. 3 (March 1, 2010): 207–27, https://doi.org/10.2165/11317090-000000000-00000.

- Tobias Engeroff, David A. Groneberg, and Jan Wilke, "After Dinner Rest a While, After Supper Walk a Mile? A Systematic Review with Meta-Analysis on the Acute Postprandial Glycemic Response to Exercise Before and After Meal Ingestion in Healthy Subjects and Patients with Impaired Glucose

Tolerance," *Sports Medicine* 53, no. 4 (January 30, 2023): 849–69, https://doi.org/10.1007/s40279-022-01808-7.

- Wen-Hui Kuan, Yi-Lang Chen, and Chao-Lin Liu, "Excretion of Ni, Pb, Cu, As, and Hg in Sweat under Two Sweating Conditions," *International Journal of Environmental Research and Public Health* 19, no. 7 (April 4, 2022): 4323, https://doi.org/10.3390/ijerph19074323.

Chapter 8

- Alanna Dorsey, LuíS De Lecea, and Kimberly J. Jennings, "Neurobiological and Hormonal Mechanisms Regulating Women's Sleep," *Frontiers in Neuroscience* 14 (January 14, 2021), https://doi.org/10.3389/fnins.2020.625397.

- Alastair Scott et al., "Improving Sleep Quality Leads to Better Mental Health: A Meta-Analysis of Randomised Controlled Trials," *Sleep Medicine Reviews* 60 (December 1, 2021): 101556, https://doi.org/10.1016/j.smrv.2021.101556.

- Alicia Núñez et al., "Smoke at Night and Sleep Worse? The Associations between Cigarette Smoking with Insomnia Severity and Sleep Duration," *Sleep Health* 7, no. 2 (April 1, 2021): 177–82, https://doi.org/10.1016/j.sleh.2020.10.006.

- Angelos Vlahoyiannis et al., "A Systematic Review, Meta-Analysis and Meta-Regression on the Effects of Carbohydrates on Sleep," *Nutrients* 13, no. 4 (April 14, 2021): 1283, https://doi.org/10.3390/nu13041283.

- Anne Marie Chang et al., "Human Responses to Bright Light of Different Durations," *The Journal of Physiology* 590, no. 13 (May 30, 2012): 3103–12, https://doi.org/10.1113/jphysiol.2011.226555.

- Ben Carter et al., "Association between Portable Screen-Based Media Device Access or Use and Sleep Outcomes," *JAMA*

Pediatrics 170, no. 12 (December 1, 2016): 1202, https://doi.org/10.1001/jamapediatrics.2016.2341.

- Brendan M. Gabriel and Juleen R. Zierath, "Circadian Rhythms and Exercise — Re-Setting the Clock in Metabolic Disease," *Nature Reviews Endocrinology* 15, no. 4 (January 17, 2019): 197–206, https://doi.org/10.1038/s41574-018-0150-x.

- "Bryan Johnson," 2021, https://www.bryanjohnson.com/.

- Carissa Gardiner et al., "The Effect of Caffeine on Subsequent Sleep: A Systematic Review and Meta-Analysis," *Sleep Medicine Reviews* 69 (June 1, 2023): 101764, https://doi.org/10.1016/j.smrv.2023.101764.

- Dandan Zheng et al., "Alcohol Consumption and Sleep Quality: A Community-Based Study," *Public Health Nutrition* 24, no. 15 (November 13, 2020): 4851–58, https://doi.org/10.1017/s1368980020004553.

- Daniela Grimaldi et al., "Strengthening Sleep–Autonomic Interaction via Acoustic Enhancement of Slow Oscillations," *SLEEP* 42, no. 5 (February 6, 2019), https://doi.org/10.1093/sleep/zsz036.

- Dorothee Fischer and Cassie J. Hilditch, "Light in Ecological Settings: Entrainment, Circadian Disruption, and Interventions," *Progress in Brain Research*, 2022, 303–30, https://doi.org/10.1016/bs.pbr.2022.04.001.

- Elise R. Facer-Childs et al., "Resetting the Late Timing of 'Night Owls' Has a Positive Impact on Mental Health and Performance," *Sleep Medicine* 60 (August 1, 2019): 236–47, https://doi.org/10.1016/j.sleep.2019.05.001.

- Frances Veronica O'Callaghan, Olav Muurlink, and Natasha Reid, "Effects of Caffeine on Sleep Quality and Daytime Functioning," *Risk Management and Healthcare Policy* 11 (December 1, 2018): 263–71, https://doi.org/10.2147/rmhp.s156404.

- Jacob L. Fulton et al., "Impact of Genetic Variability on Physiological Responses to Caffeine in Humans: A Systematic Review," *Nutrients* 10, no. 10 (September 25, 2018): 1373, https://doi.org/10.3390/nu10101373.

- Jared Minkel et al., "Sleep Deprivation Potentiates HPA Axis Stress Reactivity in Healthy Adults.," *Health Psychology* 33, no. 11 (January 1, 2014): 1430–34, https://doi.org/10.1037/a0034219.

- Jean-Philippe Chaput et al., "Sleep Timing, Sleep Consistency, and Health in Adults: A Systematic Review," *Applied Physiology, Nutrition, and Metabolism* 45, no. 10 (Suppl. 2) (October 1, 2020): S232–47, https://doi.org/10.1139/apnm-2020-0032.

- Joseph A. Hanson, and Martin R. Huecker 2. *Sleep Deprivation*, StatPearls. StatPearls Publishing (June 12, 2023).

- June C. Lo et al., "Cognitive Performance, Sleepiness, and Mood in Partially Sleep Deprived Adolescents: The Need for Sleep Study," *Sleep* 39, no. 3 (March 1, 2016): 687–98, https://doi.org/10.5665/sleep.5552.

- Konstantinos Mantantzis et al., "Effects of Dietary Carbohydrate Profile on Nocturnal Metabolism, Sleep, and Wellbeing: A Review," *Frontiers in Public Health* 10 (July 13, 2022), https://doi.org/10.3389/fpubh.2022.931781.

- Marcia Ines Silvani, Robert Werder, and Catherine Perret, "The Influence of Blue Light on Sleep, Performance and Wellbeing in Young Adults: A Systematic Review," *Frontiers in Physiology* 13 (August 16, 2022), https://doi.org/10.3389/fphys.2022.943108.

- Marie-Pierre St-Onge, Anja Mikic, and Cara E Pietrolungo, "Effects of Diet on Sleep Quality," *Advances in Nutrition* 7, no. 5 (September 1, 2016): 938–49, https://doi.org/10.3945/an.116.012336.

- Melis Yilmaz Balban et al., "Brief Structured Respiration Practices Enhance Mood and Reduce Physiological Arousal," *Cell Reports Medicine* 4, no. 1 (January 1, 2023): 100895, https://doi.org/10.1016/j.xcrm.2022.100895.

- Michael A. Smith et al., "The Physical and Psychological Health Benefits of Positive Emotional Writing: Investigating the Moderating Role of Type D (Distressed) Personality," *British Journal of Health Psychology* 23, no. 4 (June 3, 2018): 857–71, https://doi.org/10.1111/bjhp.12320.

- Michal Šmotek et al., "Evening and Night Exposure to Screens of Media Devices and Its Association with Subjectively Perceived Sleep: Should 'Light Hygiene' Be given More Attention?," *Sleep Health* 6, no. 4 (August 1, 2020): 498–505, https://doi.org/10.1016/j.sleh.2019.11.007.

- Nikola Chung et al., "Does the Proximity of Meals to Bedtime Influence the Sleep of Young Adults? A Cross-Sectional Survey of University Students," *International Journal of Environmental Research and Public Health* 17, no. 8 (April 14, 2020): 2677, https://doi.org/10.3390/ijerph17082677.

- Nina Sondrup et al., "Effects of Sleep Manipulation on Markers of Insulin Sensitivity: A Systematic Review and Meta-Analysis of Randomized Controlled Trials," *Sleep Medicine Reviews* 62 (April 1, 2022): 101594, https://doi.org/10.1016/j.smrv.2022.101594.

- Núria Sempere-Rubio, Mariam Aguas, and Raquel Faubel, "Association between Chronotype, Physical Activity, and Sedentary Behaviour: A Systematic Review," *International Journal of Environmental Research and Public Health* 19, no. 15 (August 5, 2022): 9646, https://doi.org/10.3390/ijerph19159646.

- "Oura Ring: Accurate Health Information Accessible to Everyone," Oura Ring, https://ouraring.com/.

- Panayiotis Aristotelous et al., "Effects of Controlled Dehydration on Sleep Quality and Quantity: A Polysomnographic Study in Healthy Young Adults," *Journal of Sleep Research* 28, no. 3 (February 7, 2018), https://doi.org/10.1111/jsr.12662.

- Reinoso Suárez. "Neurobiología del sueño de ondas lentas [The neurobiology of slow-wave sleep]." *Anales de la Real Academia Nacional de Medicina*, 116. (1999) (1), 209–226.

- Seth A. Creasy et al., "Effect of Sleep on Weight Loss and Adherence to Diet and Physical Activity Recommendations during an 18-Month Behavioral Weight Loss Intervention," *International Journal of Obesity* 46, no. 8 (May 16, 2022): 1510–17, https://doi.org/10.1038/s41366-022-01141-z.

- Shahab Haghayegh et al., "Before-Bedtime Passive Body Heating by Warm Shower or Bath to Improve Sleep: A Systematic Review and Meta-Analysis," *Sleep Medicine Reviews* 46 (August 1, 2019): 124–35, https://doi.org/10.1016/j.smrv.2019.04.008.

- Shahab Haghayegh et al., "Before-Bedtime Passive Body Heating by Warm Shower or Bath to Improve Sleep: A Systematic Review and Meta-Analysis," *Sleep Medicine Reviews* 46 (August 1, 2019): 124–35, https://doi.org/10.1016/j.smrv.2019.04.008.

- Stephen Parker, "Training Attention for Conscious Non-REM Sleep: The Yogic Practice of Yoga-Nidrā and Its Implications for Neuroscience Research," *Progress in Brain Research*, 2019, 255–72, https://doi.org/10.1016/bs.pbr.2018.10.016.

- Su I. Lao et al., "Associations between Bedtime Eating or Drinking, Sleep Duration and Wake after Sleep Onset: Findings from the American Time Use Survey," *British Journal of Nutrition* 127, no. 12 (September 13, 2021): 1888–97, https://doi.org/10.1017/s0007114521003597.

- Takafumi Maeda et al., "Effects of Bathing-Induced Changes in Body Temperature on Sleep," *Journal of Physiological*

Anthropology 42, no. 1 (September 8, 2023), https://doi. org/10.1186/s40101-023-00337-0.

- Yanbo Chen, "Relationship between Sleep and Muscle Strength among Chinese University Students: A Cross-Sectional Study," *Journal of Musculoskeletal & Neuronal Interactions* vol. 17,4 (December 1, 2017): 327-333. https://www.ncbi.nlm. nih.gov/pmc/articles/PMC5749041/.

Chapter 9

- 40 Years of Zen, "40 Years of Zen Neurofeedback Training - 40 Years of Zen," (September 25, 2023), https://40yearsofzen.com/.

- Alia J. Crum et al., "Evaluation of the 'Rethink Stress' Mindset Intervention: A Metacognitive Approach to Changing Mindsets.," *Journal of Experimental Psychology: General* 152, no. 9 (September 1, 2023): 2603–22, https://doi.org/10.1037/ xge0001396.

- André Schulz et al., "The Relationship between Self-Reported Chronic Stress, Physiological Stress Axis Dysregulation and Medically-Unexplained Symptoms," *Biological Psychology* 183 (October 1, 2023): 108690, https://doi.org/10.1016/j. biopsycho.2023.108690.

- Andrea Zaccaro et al., "How Breath-Control Can Change Your Life: A Systematic Review on Psycho-Physiological Correlates of Slow Breathing," *Frontiers in Human Neuroscience* 12 (September 7, 2018), https://doi.org/10.3389/fnhum.2018.00353.

- Aneeque Jamil et al., "Meditation and Its Mental and Physical Health Benefits in 2023," *Cureus*, 15,6, (June 19, 2023): e40650, https://doi.org/10.7759/cureus.40650.

- Callum Parker et al., "Does the Self-Reported Playfulness of Older Adults Influence Their Wellbeing? An Exploratory Study," *Scandinavian Journal of Occupational Therapy* 30, no. 1

(November 21, 2022): 86–97, https://doi.org/10.1080/1103812 8.2022.2145993.

- Carl J. Charnetski and Francis X. Brennan, "Sexual Frequency and Salivary Immunoglobulin A (IgA)," *Psychological Reports* 94, no. 3 (June 1, 2004): 839–44, https://doi.org/10.2466/ pr0.94.3.839-844.

- Carlotta Florentine Oesterling et al., "The Influence of Sexual Activity on Sleep: A Diary Study," *Journal of Sleep Research* 32, no. 4 (January 16, 2023), https://doi.org/10.1111/jsr.13814.

- Daniel A. Dumesic et al., "Interplay of Cortisol, Testosterone, and Abdominal Fat Mass in Normal-Weight Women with Polycystic Ovary Syndrome," *Journal of the Endocrine Society* 7, no. 8 (June 7, 2023), https://doi.org/10.1210/jendso/ bvad079.

- Dorit Haim-Litevsky, Reut Komemi, and Lena Lipskaya-Velikovsky, "Sense of Belonging, Meaningful Daily Life Participation, and Well-Being: Integrated Investigation," *International Journal of Environmental Research and Public Health* 20, no. 5 (February 25, 2023): 4121, https://doi.org/10.3390/ ijerph20054121.

- Elissa S. Epel et al., "Stress and Body Shape: Stress-Induced Cortisol Secretion Is Consistently Greater among Women with Central Fat," *Psychosomatic Medicine* 62, no. 5 (September 1, 2000): 623–32, https://doi.org/10.1097/00006842-200009000-00005.

- Eunice Y Park et al., "Sense of Community and Mental Health: A Cross-Sectional Analysis from a Household Survey in Wisconsin," *Family Medicine and Community Health* 11, no. 2 (June 1, 2023): e001971, https://doi.org/10.1136/fmch-2022-001971.

- Fariha Angum et al., "The Prevalence of Autoimmune Disorders in Women: A Narrative Review," *Cureus*, 12,5, (May 13, 2020): e8094, https://doi.org/10.7759/cureus.8094.

- Gabor Maté, *When the Body Says No: Exploring the Stress-Disease Connection* (Trade Paper Press, 2011), 320.

- Giselle Soares Passos et al., "Insomnia Severity Is Associated with Morning Cortisol and Psychological Health," *Sleep Science* 16, no. 01 (March 1, 2023): 092–096, https://doi.org/10.1055/s-0043-1767754.

- Gregory L. Fricchione, "Mind Body Medicine: A Modern Bio-Psycho-Social Model Forty-Five Years after Engel," *BioPsychoSocial Medicine* 17, no. 1 (March 30, 2023), https://doi.org/10.1186/s13030-023-00268-3.

- Guy W. Fincham et al., "Effect of Breathwork on Stress and Mental Health: A Meta-Analysis of Randomised-Controlled Trials," *Scientific Reports* 13, no. 1 (January 9, 2023), https://doi.org/10.1038/s41598-022-27247-y.

- Hanna Eilers, Marije Aan Het Rot, and Bertus F. Jeronimus, "Childhood Trauma and Adult Somatic Symptoms," *Psychosomatic Medicine* 85, no. 5 (April 26, 2023): 408–16, https://doi.org/10.1097/psy.0000000000001208.

- James Nestor, *Breath: The New Science of a Lost Art* (Riverhead Books, 2020), 304.

- Jenna Alley et al., "Associations between Oxytocin and Cortisol Reactivity and Recovery in Response to Psychological Stress and Sexual Arousal.," *Psychoneuroendocrinology* 106 (August 1, 2019): 47–56, https://doi.org/10.1016/j.psyneuen.2019.03.031.

- Jeremy Peabody et al., "A Systematic Review of Heart Rate Variability as a Measure of Stress in Medical Professionals," *Cureus*, 15,1 (January 29, 2023): e34345, https://doi.org/10.7759/cureus.34345.

- Joanna L. Spencer-Segal and Huda Akil, "Glucocorticoids and Resilience," *Hormones and Behavior* 111 (May 1, 2019): 131–34, https://doi.org/10.1016/j.yhbeh.2018.11.005.

- Joshua A. Waxenbaum, Vamsi Reddy, Matthew Varacallo, "*Anatomy, Autonomic Nervous System,*" StatPearls, StatPearls Publishing, (July 24, 2023).

- Kathryn E. Flynn et al., "Sexual Satisfaction and the Importance of Sexual Health to Quality of Life throughout the Life Course of U.S. Adults," *The Journal of Sexual Medicine* 13, no. 11 (November 1, 2016): 1642–50, https://doi.org/10.1016/j.jsxm.2016.08.011.

- Lara Lakhsassi et al., "The Influence of Sexual Arousal on Subjective Pain Intensity during a Cold Pressor Test in Women," *PLOS ONE* 17, no. 10 (October 5, 2022): e0274331, https://doi.org/10.1371/journal.pone.0274331.

- Lora M. Mullen et al., "Facilitation of Forgiveness," *Holistic Nursing Practice* 37, no. 1 (January 1, 2023): 15–23, https://doi.org/10.1097/hnp.0000000000000559.

- Marie Kuhfuß et al., "Somatic Experiencing – Effectiveness and Key Factors of a Body-Oriented Trauma Therapy: A Scoping Literature Review," *European Journal of Psychotraumatology* 12, no. 1 (January 1, 2021), https://doi.org/10.1080/20008198.2021.1929023.

- Mariesa Cay et al., "Childhood Maltreatment and Its Role in the Development of Pain and Psychopathology," *The Lancet Child & Adolescent Health* 6, no. 3 (March 1, 2022): 195–206, https://doi.org/10.1016/s2352-4642(21)00339-4.

- Melis Yilmaz Balban et al., "Brief Structured Respiration Practices Enhance Mood and Reduce Physiological Arousal," *Cell Reports Medicine* 4, no. 1 (January 1, 2023): 100895, https://doi.org/10.1016/j.xcrm.2022.100895.

- Nayak, Chetan S. and Arayamparambil C. Anilkumar. *EEG Normal Waveforms.* StatPearls, StatPearls Publishing, (July 24, 2023).

- Noa Rofe et al., "Salivary Cortisol Concentration and Perceived Stress Measure in Response to Acute Natural Stress:

The Role of Morningness-Eveningness Preference," *Chronobiology International*, (November 2, 2023), 1–7, https://doi.org/10.1080/07420528.2023.2276203.

- Olivia Pastore, Benjamin L. Brett, and Michelle Fortier, "Self-Compassion and Happiness: Exploring the Influence of the Subcomponents of Self-Compassion on Happiness and Vice Versa," *Psychological Reports* 126, no. 5 (April 15, 2022): 2191–2211, https://doi.org/10.1177/00332941221084902.

- "On My Mind: RBG, Surge Capacity, and Play as an Energy Source - Brené Brown," Brené Brown, (July 5, 2023), https://brenebrown.com/podcast/on-my-mind-rbg-surge-capacity-and-play-as-an-energy-source/.

- Regena Thomashauer, *Pussy: A Reclamation* (Hay House, 2018) 288.

- Shi-Kai Wang et al., "Psychological Trauma, Posttraumatic Stress Disorder and Trauma-Related Depression: A Mini-Review," *World Journal of Psychiatry* 13, no. 6 (June 19, 2023): 331–39, https://doi.org/10.5498/wjp.v13.i6.331.

- Stuart Brody, "Blood Pressure Reactivity to Stress Is Better for People Who Recently Had Penile–Vaginal Intercourse than for People Who Had Other or No Sexual Activity," *Biological Psychology* 71, no. 2 (February 1, 2006): 214–22, https://doi.org/10.1016/j.biopsycho.2005.03.005.

- Turhan Canli et al., "Sex Differences in the Neural Basis of Emotional Memories," *Proceedings of the National Academy of Sciences of the United States of America* 99, no. 16 (July 26, 2002): 10789–94, https://doi.org/10.1073/pnas.162356599.

- Ziva, "Sign Up For Our Free Masterclass! - Ziva," (May 31, 2023), https://zivameditation.com/freemasterclass-1/?gc_id=19655298857&h_ad_id=647406365935&gad_source=1&gclid=CjwKCAiA0syqBhBxEiwAeNx9Nyl9NnnGE4oOXVk10gTZYb3I-uy80VPpU0vHzA5WmieDYPSBpwmxr9xoCcP8QAvD_BwE.

ABOUT THE AUTHOR

Aggie Lal is a renowned public figure, best-selling author, certified nutrition and health coach, podcast host, TV personality, and TEDx speaker. With more than 1.5 million social media followers and a vast audience across multiple channels, Aggie has become highly influential in the areas of health, biohacking, personal development, entrepreneurship, and travel & lifestyle.

Her journey to success is a testament to her resilience and determination. Born in post-communist Poland, Aggie faced numerous challenges, including a life-altering car accident that left her disabled. But despite these obstacles, Aggie was determined to forge her own path rather than to be defined by her circumstances.

From sailing across the Pacific in 2012 to founding the "Travel In Her Shoes" blog that has captivated millions worldwide, Aggie built a social media presence that chronicled her discovery of a love for adventure, seizing the moment, and encouraging others to live their own very best lives.

Aggie's success has not been without its challenges, however. Determined to heal herself from depression, anxiety, and panic attacks—and to help others facing similar struggles—Aggie began to redefine her purpose and impact. Beginning with her first TEDx talk in 2019, where she shared her story of resilience and transformation, Aggie began exploring new ways of flourishing, including biohacking—the practice of optimizing one's body and mind through scientific and holistic methods.

Aggie's commitment to empowering women led her to establish the Higher Self Academy, where she has created multiple courses that have transformed the lives of over 20,000 students in the realms of health, personal development, and biohacking. Her courses, including "F*ck the Struggle," "Fit As F*ck," "10-Day Hormone Challenge," and "The Anti-Aging Challenge," empower women to tap into their highest potential, achieve their health goals, and reverse the aging process. Her Biohacking Bestie™ line of supplements are formulated by some of the world's leading experts in biohacking technology and nutrition. Her podcast, also called *Biohacking Bestie*, features conversations with many of the most prominent voices in the health and wellness industry today, as well as interviews with experts on psychiatry, brain health, and personal development.

As a natural presenter and speaker, Aggie has promoted personal health and joyful living in TV appearances around the globe such as *Dancing With the Stars*, and many more.

Today, Aggie is a visionary biohacker, empowering millennial and Gen Z women globally to optimize their health, fitness, and overall well-being. With a decade-long social media presence as one of the first viral creatives on Instagram and over 1.5 million followers across platforms to date, she inspires women to live abundant, fulfilling lives with a holistic perspective grounded in mindfulness and spirituality.

Aggie's first book, *Instatravel*, is a worldwide bestseller that chronicles her extraordinary travels and experiences as a renowned travel personality. *Biohack Like a Woman* is her second book, and delves into the world of biohacking from a uniquely female perspective by providing invaluable insights for optimizing health and well-being in routines and practices maximized for women's bodies. With her dedication to holistic well-being, Aggie Lal is at the forefront of empowering women to optimize their health and thrive in all areas of life.

Find Aggie at:

https://www.instagram.com/aggie/
https://www.instagram.com/biohackingbestie/
https://higherselfacademy.co/
https://biohackingbestie.com/

FREE WORKOUT AND MEAL PLAN

You made it! Or maybe you skipped to the end . . . but either way, we at Biohacking Bestie ™ have a special gift for you.

Go here and chat with an Artificial Intelligence Aggie.
Wait—what?
That's right! An AI Aggiebot is waiting to engage with all your biohacking questions and to offer personalized guidance.